Sameh Mezri

Results of combined treatment of lymph node tuberculosis

Sameh Mezri

Results of combined treatment of lymph node tuberculosis

ScienciaScripts

Imprint
Any brand names and product names mentioned in this book are subject to trademark, brand or patent protection and are trademarks or registered trademarks of their respective holders. The use of brand names, product names, common names, trade names, product descriptions etc. even without a particular marking in this work is in no way to be construed to mean that such names may be regarded as unrestricted in respect of trademark and brand protection legislation and could thus be used by anyone.

Cover image: www.ingimage.com

This book is a translation from the original published under ISBN 978-613-8-46940-7.

Publisher:
Sciencia Scripts
is a trademark of
Dodo Books Indian Ocean Ltd. and OmniScriptum S.R.L publishing group

120 High Road, East Finchley, London, N2 9ED, United Kingdom
Str. Armeneasca 28/1, office 1, Chisinau MD-2012, Republic of Moldova, Europe
Printed at: see last page
ISBN: 978-620-4-11909-0

Table of contents:

List of abbreviations

ACFA: Atrial fibrillation arrhythmia.

FDC : Fixed-dose combinations of anti-tuberculosis chemotherapy.

ALAT: Alanine Amino Transferase.

ASAT: Aspartate Amino-Transferase.

BCG: Bacillus Calmette and Guerin.

BK: Koch's bacillus.

CMF: Surgery-maxillofacial.

DDT: start of treatment.

DOTS: Directly Observed Short course of Treatment.

AE: Adverse Effect.

GG: Ganglionic.

GGT: Gamma Glutamyl-Transferase.

HR: Isoniazid-Rifampicin.

HRZ: Isoniazid-Rifampicin-Pyrazinamide.

HRZE: Isoniazid-Rifampicin-Pyrazinamide-Ethambutol.

HTA: High blood pressure.

TST: Tuberculin Intradermal Reaction.

INH: Isoniazid.

CKD: chronic renal failure.

JC: Jugulo-carotid.

No.: Number.

CBC: Blood Count.

Nle: Normal.

NORB: Retrobulbar Optic Neuritis.

WHO: World Health Organization.

ENT: Ear, Nose and Throat.

PAL: Alkaline phosphatase.

PNLT: National Tuberculosis Control Programme.

TAP: Thoracic-Abdomino-Pelvic.

CT: Computed tomography.

PET: Extra-Pulmonary Tuberculosis.

Ttt: Treatment.

HIV: Human Immunodeficiency Virus.

INTRODUCTION

Tuberculosis remains a major global health problem and TB control is a priority for WHO.

Tunisia is a country with intermediate endemicity with an incidence of 30/100,000 inhabitants in 2012 [1]. However, there is an upsurge in extra-pulmonary forms, particularly lymph nodes, which account for more than 50% of these localizations. Cervical localization represents 70 to 90% of all lymph node forms [2].

The main challenge of national programmes is to obtain the best cure rate by improving adherence to treatment and reducing the rate of resistant forms. For this reason, several procedures have been proposed such as free treatment and the DOTS strategy "directly observed short course of treatment". In addition to these methods, Tunisia has introduced since July 2009 the fixed-dose combinations of anti-tuberculosis chemotherapy (ADF) or combined forms, in accordance with the recommendations of the national program of the fight against tuberculosis (PNLT).

These combinations have facilitated prescribing for the practitioner and improved compliance for the patient. The aim is to avoid incomplete use of the separate antibiotics and thus the risk of selection of resistant strains [3]. However, few studies have assessed the therapeutic results of these combined forms and identified their shortcomings.

Through our study, we propose:

- To evaluate the therapeutic results of ADFs in the treatment of cervical lymph node tuberculosis in terms of cure, relapse and adverse effects.
- Identify factors that have influenced our treatment outcomes.
- Propose a therapeutic attitude in front of a tuberculous adenopathy according to the clinical presentation.

PATIENTS AND METHODS

I- PATIENTS :

I-1- Type of study :

This is a retrospective descriptive longitudinal study of patients who were managed at the ENT and CMF department of the Tunis Military Hospital for cervical lymph node tuberculosis and who were treated with the combined form of antituberculosis chemotherapy.

I-2- Patient selection :

I-2-1- Inclusion criteria :

We included patients over 16 years of age, treated for cervical lymph node tuberculosis, who were prescribed anti-tuberculosis chemotherapy in its combined form (**HRZE/HR**) since its introduction in the department, i.e. the period from July 2009 to May 2016. A minimum setback of 6 months after the end of treatment was required.

I-2-2- Exclusion criteria :

The following were excluded from this study:

- Patients under 16 years of age (pediatric population).
- Patients with missing data in their records.
- Patients treated with the dissociated form from the start.
- Patients who have never attended the postoperative medical check-up.
- Patients who have not completed a full course of treatment.
- Patients correctly followed up but less than 6 months after the end of treatment.

I-3- Diagnostic confirmation :

Treatment was prescribed after diagnostic confirmation obtained in all cases by **histological study of** surgical biopsies of cervical adenopathies.

I-4- Pre-therapeutic assessment :

Prior to initiation of anti-tuberculosis treatment, all patients underwent a pre-treatment workup including:

- A weighing of the patient in order to adapt the dosage.
- Chest x-ray.
- A specialized ophthalmological examination with a visual field study, a color vision test and a fundus.
- A measurement of hearing acuity using baseline pure tone audiometry.
- A sputum BK test on 3 consecutive days to look for an unlabeled pulmonary location on the

chest X-ray.

- A biological assessment with study:
    1. Liver function (ASAT, ALAT, GGT, PAL, Bilirubin).
    2. Renal function (Urea, creatinine clearance).
    3. Uric acid determination, blood ionogram.
    4. A haematological check-up (CBC, platelets).
- An isoniazid acetylation test that was performed for 23 patients (46%).

It should be noted that patients who were not treated with the combined form of anti-tuberculosis antibiotic therapy were excluded from the study from the start.

I-5- Therapeutic protocol :

As soon as the diagnosis was confirmed, all our patients were put on effective dose antituberculosis chemotherapy in combined form according to the scheme recommended by the strategy of the National Tuberculosis Control Programme (NTCP) which is adapted to the patient's weight (Table I).

Table I: Dosages of combined anti-tuberculosis treatment according to weight for adults

	30-39kg	40-55 kg	55-70 kg	>70kg
HRZE (75mg+150mg+400mg+275mg)	2cp	3cp	4cp	5cp
HR (75mg+150mg)	2cp	3cp	4cp	5cp

I-6- Monitoring under treatment :

Monitoring was clinical, biological and ultrasound:

- Clinical: weight gain, tolerance of treatment, possible side effects, examination of lymph nodes.
  A first check-up was planned at 21 days (on average) of treatment, then at 2, 4, 6, 9 and 12 months and at 6 months after the end of treatment. Subsequently, the follow-up rate was scheduled on a case-by-case basis.
  Specialized examinations, particularly ophthalmological ones, were indicated in case of suspected adverse effects or pathological initial examination.
- Biological: concomitant to the clinical control with the practice of a haemogram, a hepatic assessment, a uricemia and a renal assessment.
- Ultrasound: systematic at the end of the treatment. An ultrasound check-up was also requested when new adenopathies appeared and/or their size increased.

I-7- Criteria for treatment effectiveness :

Given the lack of clear consensus on the definition of treatment outcome in lymph node TB, we used the definitions proposed in the Tunisian TB management guide 2014 (Table II).

Table II: Definition of patient status at the end of treatment

Cure	Absence of any signs of clinical and/or ultrasound at the end of the treatment
Treatment failure	Clinical and/or radiological persistence of evolution of pre-existing adenopathies or appearance of new adenopathies
Recidivism	Increase in size of a residual lymph node or appearance of one or more lymph nodes after a complete cure and clinical remission phase
Deaths	Death during treatment (any cause)
Treatment interrupted	Treatment interrupted for 2 months or more before scheduled completion or not completed on time
Treatment completed	Treatment completed without bacteriological evidence

There is no consensus as to when these statuses for lymph node TB should be defined. Therefore, we have defined failure by the absence of decrease and/or increase in the size of adenopathies and/or the appearance of new adenopathies or productive fistulas after 9 months of treatment.

11. METHODS:

II-1- Data collection :

We proceeded to the exploitation of the patients' files thanks to a pre-established computerized form studying the epidemiological parameters, the functional signs, the data of the clinical and para-clinical examinations, the therapeutic protocol, the follow-up, the evolution during the treatment and the possible complications related to the treatment or to the disease (Appendix 1)

II-2- Statistical methods :

- Data entry :

The data collected was computerized using the statistical computer program: SPSS 17.

- Descriptive study :

Simple frequencies and relative frequencies (percentages) were calculated for the categorical variables. Quantitative variables were expressed as averages and qualitative variables as proportions.

II-3- Bibliographic research :

We used the websites PUBMED, Springer Link and Science Direct to search for bibliographic references using the following keywords: lymph node tuberculosis, combined anti-tuberculosis drugs, therapeutic protocol, results, therapeutics.

II-4- Ethical considerations and conflicts of interest :

In our retrospective and descriptive work, data collection was carried out from medical records and was not conditional on the prior consent of the patients included.

We declare that we have no personal conflicts of interest that are incompatible with the objectives of this work.

RESULTS

I- EPIDEMIOLOGICAL STUDY :

I-1- Incidence of tuberculosis :

During the study period, we collected 50 cases of cervical lymph node tuberculosis diagnosed and treated with the combined form of anti-tuberculosis drugs at the ENT and CMF department of the Tunis Military Hospital. A peak in frequency was noted in 2013 and 2015 with an average of seven new cases per year (Figure 1).

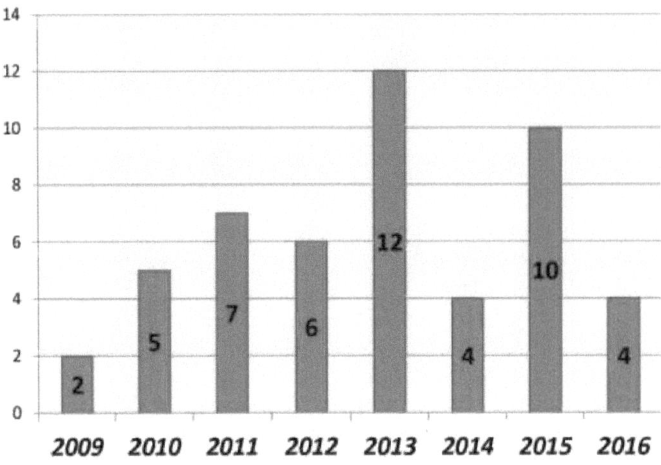

Figure 1: Distribution of patients by year

This incidence is certainly higher because of the exclusion of patients treated with the dissociated form of anti-tuberculosis drugs.

I-2- Age :

The mean age of our patients was 34 years with extremes of 17 and 78 years. Fifty percent of the cases were young adults [20-40 years] and 18% were less than 20 years old at diagnosis (Figure 2).

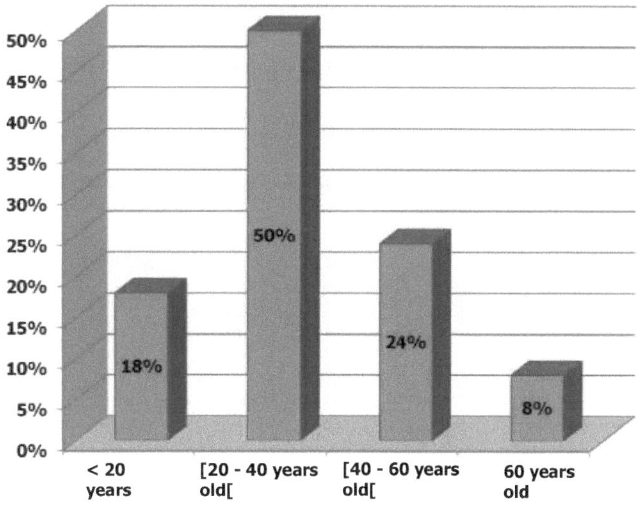

Figure 2: Age distribution of patients

I-3- Sex :

There was no gender predominance in our series, with 26 female patients (52%) and 24 male patients (48%) (Figure 3).

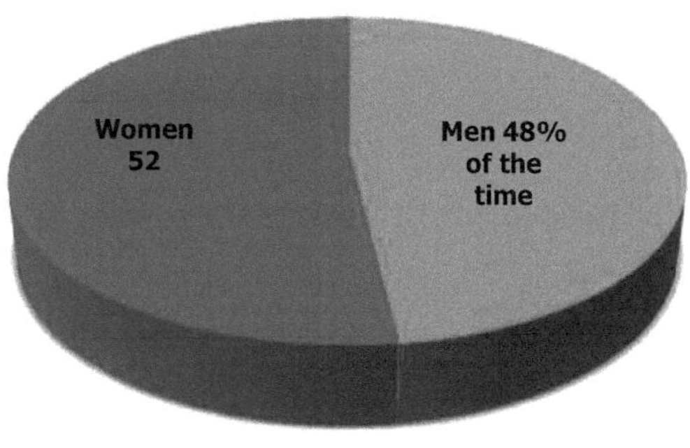

Figure 3: Gender distribution of patients

I-4- Place of residence :

Twenty-five patients (50% of the cases) resided in the greater Tunis area, 52% in the governorate of Tunis and 36% in Mannouba (Figure 4).

The notion of living in a community was reported by 7 patients (14%).

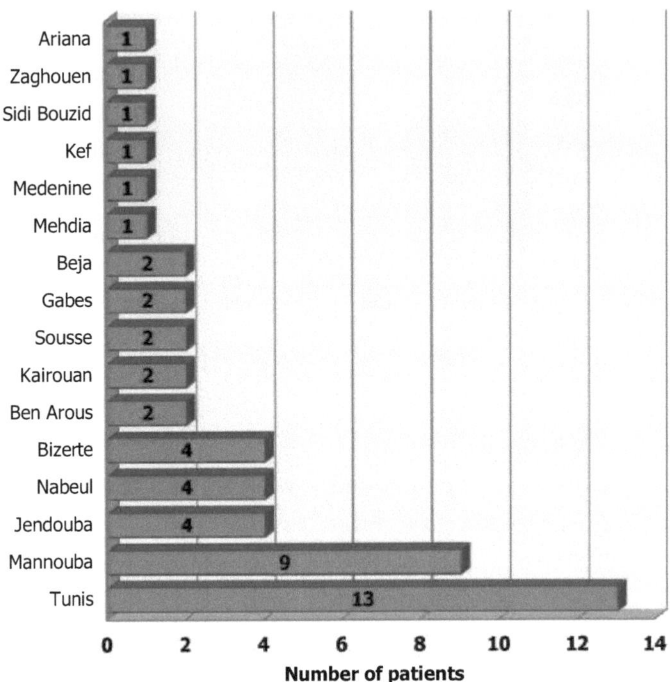

Figure 4: Distribution of patients by origin

I-5- Profession :

Occupation was specified in only 35 cases. The patients were most often of middle class social status (Table III).

Table III: Distribution of patients by occupation

Profession	Number of cases	Percentage
Career Military	9	18%
Housewife	10	20%
Pupil/Student	9	18%
Seamstress	1	2%
Health personnel	1	2%
Farmer	5	10%
Not specified	15	30%

II- CLINICAL STUDY :

II-1- Interrogation :

II-1-1- BCG vaccination status :

It was only specified in 20 patients (40%) of whom only 14 reported correct vaccination.

II-1-2- History of tuberculosis :

- Four patients (8%) had a history of treated and cured tuberculosis, two of which were in the cervical lymph nodes, one in the digestive tract and one in the lungs.

- The notion of contact with a tuberculosis patient (in the family or in the entourage) was reported by four patients (8% of cases). Three of these patients had pulmonary tuberculosis and one had lymph node tuberculosis.

II-1-3- Habits :

The consumption of unpasteurized raw dairy products was reported by 28 patients (56%). These were mainly cottage cheese and fermented milk.

II-1-4- Co-morbidity :

The main associated pathologies were immunodepressive diseases with one case of Behçet's disease and one case of asthma under long-term general corticosteroid therapy as well as two cases of diabetes (Figure 5).

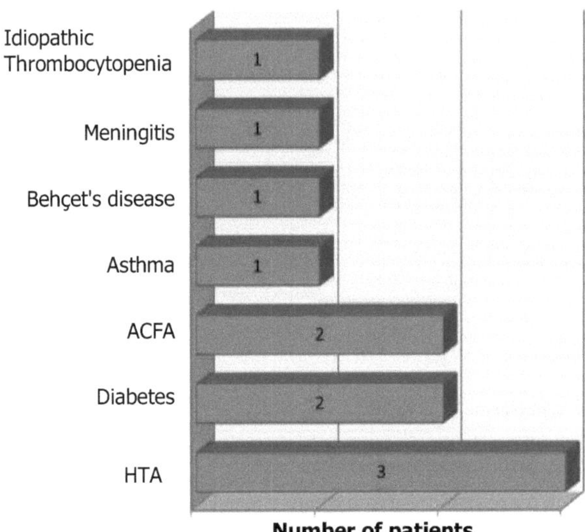

Figure 5: Distribution of patient's medical history

II-1-5- Circumstances of discovery :

All patients consulted for the finding of chronic cervical swelling. The mean time to progression of the symptomatology was 6.9 months with extremes of 1 month and 4 years (Figure 6).

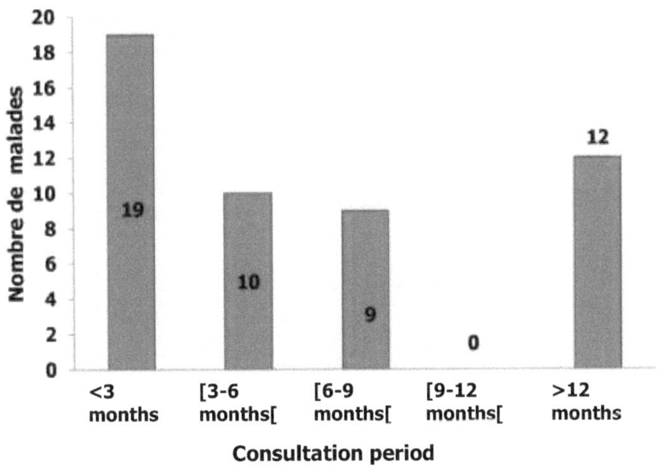

Figure 6: Distribution of Patients by Time to Consultation

II-1-6- Signs of tuberculosis impregnation :

Signs of tuberculosis impregnation were reported by 19 patients (38%). Asthenia and weight loss were the most frequently reported signs (Table IV).

Table IV: Distribution of signs of tuberculosis impregnation

	Fever	Weight loss	Asthenia	Night sweats	No signs
Number of cases	9	12	12	7	31
Percentage	18%	24%	24%	14%	62%

II-2- Physical examination :

The clinical examination was performed systematically, including an examination of all lymph nodes and a complete ENT examination, with particular emphasis on nasal endoscopy.

II-2-1- Clinical characteristics of cervical adenopathy :

II-2-1-1- Headquarters :

- The jugulo-carotid chain (JC) was the most affected; 50% of patients had group III adenopathies and 36% group IIa (Figure 7).

- The involvement was bilateral in 18 cases (36%).

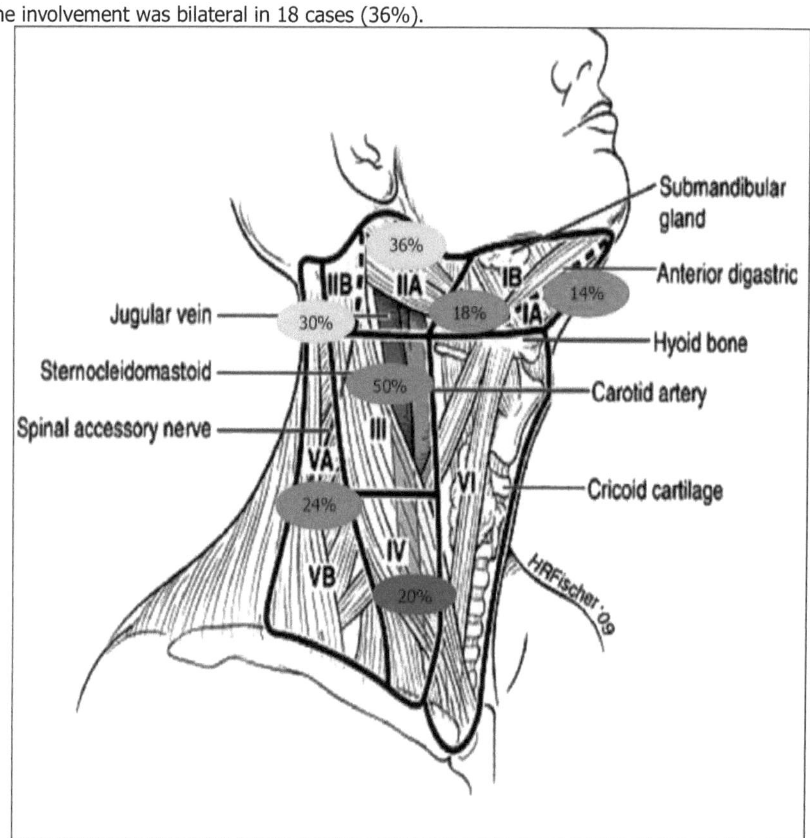

Figure 7: Sites of adenopathy

II-2-1-2- Number :

Sixty-eight percent of the patients (34 cases) had multiple adenopathies at the time of diagnosis while 16 patients (32%) had a single adenopathy.

II-2-1-3- Size :

Adenopathies had a mean size of 2.9 cm with extremes of 0.5 cm and 7 cm.

II-2-1-4- Consistency :

The consistency was hard in 2 cases and renitent in 3 cases.

In the remaining cases, the adenopathies were firm in consistency.

II-2-1-5- Mobility :

Forty-one patients (82%) had mobile adenopathies in relation to both the superficial and deep planes. In 9 cases (18%), the adenopathies were fixed.

II-2-1-6-Aspect of the skin opposite the adenopathy:

We noted fistulization to the skin in 5 patients (10%) and inflammatory skin in 4 patients (8%). In the other cases, the skin was healthy.

II-2-2- Rest of the ENT examination :

In total, we noted irregular thickening of the cavum in 3 patients (whose biopsy confirmed tuberculosis in 2 cases) and a non-surgical thyroid goiter in one case.

II-2-3- Rest of the physical examination :

One patient had inguinal adenopathy with recent alteration of general condition.

II-3- Radiological examinations :

II-3-1- Cervical ultrasound :

When a cervical swelling was observed, all patients were investigated by a cervical ultrasound scan which showed multiple adenopathies in 80% of cases (40 cases).

The echogenicity of the adenopathies was specified in 47 files with a predominance of hypoechogenic (47%) and necrotic (41%) appearance (Table V).

Table V: Ultrasound characteristics of adenopathy

		Number	Percentage (%)
Adenopathy	Unique	10	20%
	Multiple	40	80%
Size	Minimal	0.5 cm	
	Maximum	5 cm	
	Average	1.9 cm	
Ultrasound appearance (47 cases)	Hypoechogenic/heterogeneous	22	47%
	Hypoechogenic/Hyperechogenic	4	8%
	Necrosis	19	41%
	Calcification	2	4%

II-3-2- Chest X-ray :

It was performed in all patients and revealed an enlarged mediastinum in one case.

II-3-3- Other radiological investigations :

- Nine patients were investigated by cervical computed tomography (CT) in the presence of a clinically suspicious appearance of the cavum and/or adenopathy larger than 3 cm and/or attached to the superficial and deep planes (Figure 8).

- Among three patients who had a thoracoabdomino-pelvic CT scan, one patient had a magma of deep mediastinal, retroperitoneal and pelvic adenopathies. The request for a CT scan was indicated in cases of resistance to treatment and in the context of a search for deep adenopathy.

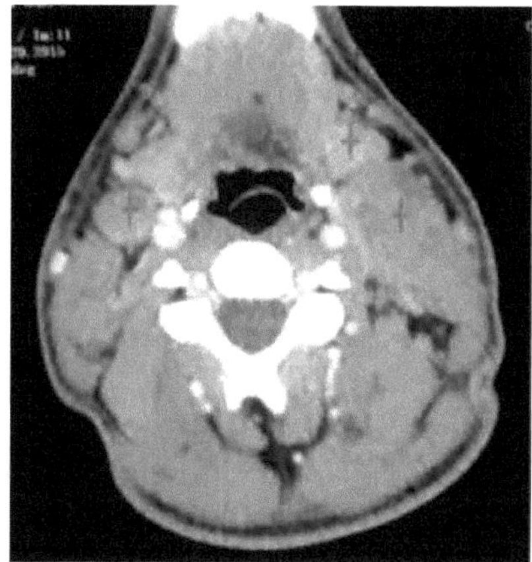

Figure 8: Cervical CT scan showing bilateral globular and necrotic cervical adenopathy (

Table VI summarizes the different CT aspects of adenopathy:

Table VI: Scannographic appearance of adenopathy

Aspect		Number
Density	Hypodense	1
	Heterogeneous	3
	Necrosis	5
Relationship to the vascular axis	Adhesion	4

II-4- Positive diagnosis :

II-4-1- Diagnostic examination :

- Intradermal tuberculin test :

In our study, the purified tuberculin intradermal test was performed in 44 patients (88%). It was positive (diameter >10 mm at 72 hours) in 39 patients (78%), of whom 12 had a phlyctenular TST. Elsewhere, 5 patients had a negative TST (10%) (Figure 9).

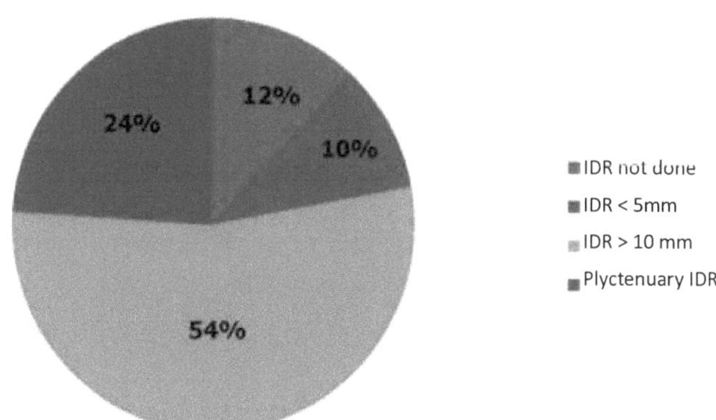

Figure 9: Intradermal results

II-4-2- Bacteriological examinations :

II-4-2-1- Search for BK in lymph node puncture :

Koch's bacillus (BK) was detected in the lymph node puncture fluid of 11 patients (22%). It was negative in all cases.

II-4-2-2- Search for BK in the lymph node shred :

BK testing in the lymph node shred was performed in 13 patients (26%). Direct examination was positive in one case. Culture on Lowenstein medium was negative in 5 cases (10%).

II-4-3- Cyto-histological examinations :

II-4-3-1- Cytopuncture of lymph nodes :

Node cytopuncture was performed in 11 patients (22%) and was consistent with the diagnosis of tuberculosis in 5 cases (10%), showing epithelioid and giganto-cellular granuloma with caseous necrosis. It suggested a tumoral origin in one case (Table VII).

Table VII: Cytopuncture results

Not done	78%
In favour of tuberculosis	10%
Reactionary	6%
Inconclusive	4%
Suspected malignancy	2%

II-4-3-2- Pathological examination :

All patients had surgical biopsy of cervical adenopathies with:

- 47 adenectomies (94%).
- 3 biopsies of the edges of fistulized adenopathies (6%).

Pathological examination confirmed the diagnosis of lymph node tuberculosis in all cases by showing caseo-follicular necrosis with epithelioid and giganto-cellular granuloma.

III- TREATMENT :

III-1- Pre-therapeutic assessment :

- Biological tests were normal in all patients, except for an iron deficiency anemia in one case, which did not contraindicate treatment.

- Despite an initial pathological ophthalmological examination (4 cases of dyschromatopsia and one case of diabetic retinopathy), the patients were put on the combined form of anti-tuberculosis drugs (HRZE) with a specialized clinical check-up every 15 days for the first two months of treatment.

- HIV serology was performed on a patient with extra-cervical adenopathy and general deterioration, which came back negative.

- Sputum was tested for Koch's bacillus on three consecutive days in 29 patients (58%). Direct examination and culture on Lowenstein medium were negative in all cases.

III-2- Medical treatment :

III-2-1- Antibiotic therapy for tuberculosis :

- The usual treatment regimen is two months of quadruple therapy (HRZE) followed by six to seven months of dual therapy (HR).

- For quadruple therapy, an exception was made in 6 cases. Thus the duration was :
  - Shortened to **1 month** for 3 patients, two of whom had dyschromatopsia on initial examination.
  - Extended to **3 months** in one case.
  - Extended for **4 months** for 2 patients (Table VIII).

Table VIII: Duration of Quadruple Therapy (HRZE)

Duration HRZE	Number of cases	Cause		What to do
1 month	3	Aggravation of dyschromatopsia	1 case	- Shaped passage combined HR (clinical improvement)
		Hepatic cytolysis: transaminases > 6Nle	1 case	- Dissociated form
		NORB+Allergy INH+cytolysis (transaminases < 3Nle)	1 case	- Dissociated form
2 months	44			
3 months	1	Paradoxical reaction at 6 weeks of treatment		
4 months	2	Non-compliance	1 case	
		Non-compliance+Paradoxical reaction at 2 months of treatment	1 case	

> The average duration of dual therapy was 6.9 months with a minimum of 4 months and a maximum of 16 months. It depended essentially on the clinical evolution and compliance to treatment.

> The total duration of treatment varied from 6 to 18 months with an average of 9.1 months (Figure 10). It was longer than 9 months in 15 cases (Figure 11).

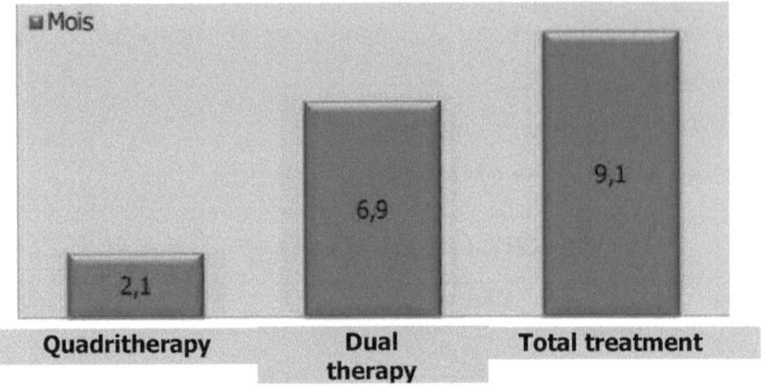

Figure 10: Average duration of TB treatment

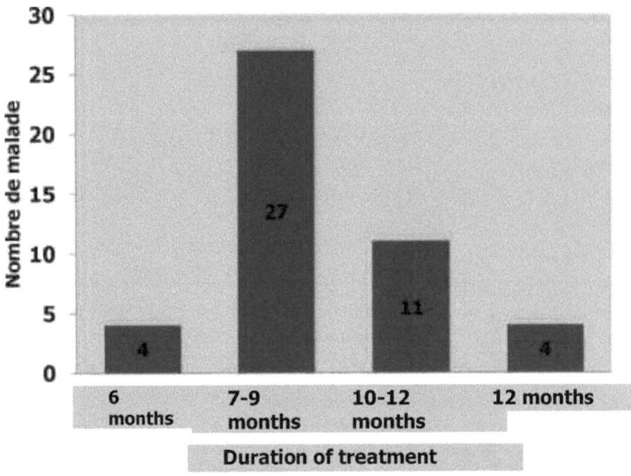

Figure 11: Distribution of patients by total duration of treatment

Overall, adherence was good in 40 cases (80%). However, adherence to treatment was better during the dual therapy period (91% versus 76% during the quadruple therapy period).

III-2-2- Evolution under treatment :

III-2-2-1- Adverse reactions :

During treatment, 26 patients (52% of cases) experienced one or more adverse events related to one of the antibiotics in the combination.

III-2-2-2- During treatment with quadritherapy (HRZE) :

- Under HRZE, 11 patients reported one or more complaints. These were mainly digestive disorders such as gastralgia and nausea. Elsewhere, they were visual disorders or allergic manifestations (Table IX).

  The severity of some of these complications led us to discontinue the combined form of treatment and switch to dissociated antibiotics in two cases and to shorten the duration of the quadritherapy in another case.

- One patient developed severe thrombocytopenia secondary to pyrazinamide at the end of the second month of treatment. Therefore, we kept the combined form of the dual therapy.

Table IX: Side effects on HRZE quadruple therapy

Adverse effect		**Number of cases (%)**
Visual disorders	Dyschromatopsia	1 (2%)
	NORB	1 (2%)
	Visual blur	3 (6%)
Allergic manifestations	Urticaria	2 (including 1 allergy to INH)
	Acne	1 (2%)
Hepatotoxicity	Transaminases < 3 Nle	4 (8%)
	Transaminases > 6 Nle	1 (2%)
Digestive disorders	Epigastralgia	9 (18%)
	Nausea	6 (12%)
	Vomiting	2 (4%)
Peripheral neuropathy		1 (2%)
Symptomatic hyperuricemia		1 (2%)
Thrombocytopenia		1 (2%)

III -2-2-3- During treatment with dual therapy (HR) :

Forty-eight patients were placed on fixed-dose dual therapy (HR), of whom 19 reported adverse events with a predominance of digestive complaints. Elsewhere, a complication was discovered during clinical and/or biological monitoring (Table X).

Table X: Side effects of dual HR therapy

Adverse effect		**Number of cases (%)**
Digestive disorders	Epigastralgia	6 (12%)
	Nausea	3 (6%)
	Vomiting	0
Hyperuricemia	Symptomatic	1 (2%)
	Biological	2 (4%)
Hepatotoxicity	Transaminases <3Nle	4 (8%)
	4-5Nle	1 (2%)
	>6Nle	1 (2%)
	Cholestasis	1(2%)
Allergic manifestations	Generalized hives	1 (2%)

- On dual therapy, one patient developed cholestasis with signs of delayed hypersensitivity (during the 5th month of treatment) which was attributed to rifampicin. A second patient developed significant hepatic cytolysis. In both cases, it was decided to stop the combined form of the drug and to switch to dissociated antibiotics and to adjust the isoniazid doses according to the acetylation test.

- Elsewhere, digestive disorders were the most reported.

III-2-3- Therapeutic evolution :

As detailed in the patients and methods chapter and to judge the effectiveness of medical treatment, we used the concepts defined in the 2014 Tunisian TB management guide.

It is important to remember that only patients who have completed a full treatment course with a minimum of 6 months after the end of treatment were included in the study.

III-2-3-1- Healing:

- Among 46 patients who had a total cure with ADF, 40 were declared cured (87% of cases).

- For these patients, the adenopathies disappeared (23 cases) or became clinically insignificant (17 cases). On follow-up ultrasound, when they still existed, they were non-specific.

- Forty patients were cured by medical treatment without recourse to other therapeutic alternatives, with variable delays; the duration of treatment was greater than 12 months in 5 cases.

III-2-3-2- Therapeutic failure :

- The failure rate for medical treatment in our series was 13% (6 cases) with persistence and/or appearance of new adenopathies of significant size clinically and radiologically after 9 months of well conducted medical treatment.

- A combination of other anti-tuberculosis drugs with or without surgery was started with good progress in all cases. The therapeutic decision as well as the monitoring were ensured in collaboration with the infectious diseases physicians.

III-2-3-3- Paradoxical reaction :

Three patients showed a paradoxical reaction:

- Two cases during HRZE treatment requiring an extension of the attack phase.
- A case at the 5th month of well conducted anti-tuberculosis treatment with significant increase in the size of adenopathies, some of which fistulated to the skin. Anti-tuberculosis treatment was maintained with a combination of corticosteroid therapy and ofloxacin for 2 months followed by surgical removal. The total duration of treatment was 18 months. The subsequent evolution was satisfactory.

III-2-3-4- Relapse :

- After being declared cured, two patients had a recurrence of their lymph node TB disease. The time to clinical remission was 6 and 12 months respectively.

- Recurrence was confirmed by histological study of an adenectomy specimen in one case and on the product of a unilateral functional lymph node dissection in the other case. The patients were put back on antituberculosis drugs: in the combined form in one case with ofloxacin and in the dissociated form in the other case.

III-3- Surgical treatment :

- Surgical treatment was decided for therapeutic purposes in eight cases (12%) (Table XI).

- For all operated patients, the total duration of treatment was greater than or equal to 9 months [9-18 months].

Table XI: Surgical management: indication and nature of the procedure

Patient	Indication	Date % DDT	Act
Female, 21 years old	Persistence of adenopathy, some of which is pre-fistulization	8 months	unilateral functional curage
Female, 22 years old	Late paradoxical reaction resistant to medical treatment	9 months	Flattening (adenectomy impossible)
Woman, 35 years old	Therapeutic failure	9 months	Right functional curing and left picking nodes
Female, 17 years old	Poor compliance	3 months	Bilateral functional curing
Male, 22 years old	Therapeutic failure	12 months	Adenectomy
Woman, 29 years old	Resistance with fistulization not responding to other anti-tuberculosis drugs	5 months	Unilateral functional curing
Female, 31 years old	Recidivism	6 months of remission	Unilateral functional curing
Male, 42 years old	Recidivism	12 months of remission	Adenectomy

- No complications related to the surgery were observed, the evolution was favorable for all patients and they were eventually declared cured.

- Pathological examination confirmed tuberculosis in all cases.

III-4- Special cases :

Three patients became pregnant during treatment. Two were beyond six months of treatment, the malformative risk was considered low and they continued their dual therapy as normal.

For the third patient, the pregnancy was discovered during the first month of treatment and a therapeutic interruption of the pregnancy was carried out after a multidisciplinary opinion (pharmacovigilance, gynaecologists).

No modification of the protocol was recommended in case of association of nasopharyngeal localization of tuberculosis. The evolution was good in both cases.

IV- FACTORS OF BAD EVOLUTION :

We tried to identify the factors associated with a poor evolution in our series (failure, resistance, relapse, need for a treatment of more than 9 months and/or surgery). Thus, we noted that:

Epidemiological factors :

> Adverse events were more frequently reported by the younger population. Thus, 77% were under 30 years of age and 4 patients between 21 and 27 years of age were recommended to switch to the dissociated form.

> With the exception of one patient aged 41 years, all patients with difficult management (surgery and/or treatment longer than 9 months) were under 30 years of age (including two under 20 years of age).

> All patients who required medical treatment for more than 9 months were female.

> Of the patients who required a combination of surgical management, only one was male (17%).

> Neither community living nor occupation was significantly correlated with worse outcomes.

Clinical factors :

> The delay in consultation did not affect the therapeutic outcome.

> Two patients with a history of treated cervical lymph node tuberculosis required a 12 and 13 month cure with functional curage in one case.

> Among five patients classified as immunocompromised, only one case (20%), had presented a clinical worsening under anti-tuberculosis drugs. On the other hand, among the cases with a bad evolution, only one was immunocompromised.

> The presence of signs of tuberculosis impregnation was no more likely to result in a poor outcome (24%).

> All patients had multiple adenopathies. Bilaterality was more frequently associated with a poor outcome (72% of cases).

Radiological factors :

> All adenopathies had a liquefied (necrotic) appearance on ultrasound.

- Seventeen patients (34%) had adenopathies larger than 3 cm. Forty-one percent of them (7 cases) had a poor evolution. On the other hand, among 11 poor evolutions, 7 (64%) had adenopathies of initial size greater than 3 cm.

- Adherence to the vascular axis of the neck (4 cases) was consistently associated with difficult management.

DISCUSSION

1- REMINDER OF THE MAIN RESULTS OF OUR STUDY :

Our study included 50 patients managed in our department for histologically confirmed cervical lymph node tuberculosis and treated with fixed-dose antituberculosis drugs during the period from July 2009 to May 2016.

- The average age of our patients was 34 years with a predominance of young adults (50% of cases). No gender predominance was noted.

    - All patients consulted because of a chronic laterocervical swelling.
    - Four patients had a history of tuberculosis, two of which were cervical lymph nodes, one pulmonary and one digestive. The notion of immunodepression was noted in five cases.
    - On clinical examination, the jugulocarotid chain was the most affected (more than 50%). The average size of the adenopathies was 2.9 cm. These were multiple in 68% of cases and bilateral in 36% of cases. Fistulization to the skin was noted in 5 cases.

- All patients were explored by cervical ultrasound. Hypoechoic appearance with heterogeneous centre was the most described (47%).

The CT scan showed extra-cervical lymph node involvement in one case and adhesion to the vascular axis in 4 cases.

- Diagnosis was confirmed by histopathological study with or without bacteriological study on biopsy-exeresis specimen. A nasopharyngeal tuberculosis location was associated in two cases.

- Before starting anti-tuberculosis antibiotic therapy, a pre-treatment assessment, as recommended by the NTP, was carried out in all patients.

    - Five patients whose initial ophthalmological examination was pathological (four cases of dyschromatopsia and one case of diabetic retinopathy) were put on combined treatment (HRZE) with close specialized clinical monitoring.

    - Our treatment regimen followed that recommended by WHO and NTP with two months of quadritherapy (HRZE) followed by four to six months of dual therapy (HR). However, the first phase of treatment was shortened to one month in three cases and extended to three or four months in three cases. The total duration of treatment was on average 9.1 months with extremes of 6 and 18 months

Monitoring was clinical, biological and ultrasound:

- With HRZE, we noted 30 adverse events reported by 11 patients.
- Under dual therapy (HR), 20 complaints were reported by 19 patients.
- In both phases, gastric disorders were prevalent.
- The main complications were ocular (NORB, dyschromatopsia) and allergic (isoniazid/rifampicin).

These events led us to discontinue the combined form and switch to the dissociated form of the anti-tuberculosis drugs in four cases.

> Among 46 patients who underwent a complete cure with ADF, 40 were declared cured (87%), five of whom had received more than 12 months of medical treatment.
> For the other cases, we associated anti-tuberculosis drugs of other families, corticosteroid therapy and/or surgical management in six cases with lateral lymph node removal in four cases.
> A paradoxical reaction was noted in three patients.

After being declared cured, two patients presented a recurrence of their tuberculosis after six and 12 months of clinical remission (4%).

> We tried to identify the factors associated with poor outcome under ADF treatment; thus, we found some:

- **Epidemiological factors:** age under 30 years and female gender.
- **Clinical factors:** presence of multiple and/or bilateral lymph nodes.
- **Radiological factors:** Adenopathy larger than 3 cm, liquefied, adherent to the vascular axis.

II- WEAKNESS AND STRENGTH OF OUR STUDY :

> Our work is a retrospective study. The retrospective nature of the study meant that some data could not be collected.

> The relatively small number of patients. Thus, a statistical study was not possible.

> The lack of a consensus on the management of lymph node tuberculosis meant that the duration of treatment, the rate of monitoring, and the definition of progression status under treatment were not codified and consistent among all physicians.

But

> Selection bias is minimized by including patients who have completed a full course of combined TB treatment with strict inclusion criteria and a 100% participation rate at six months after completion of treatment.

> Collaboration between the ENT department and the infectious diseases department has made it possible to improve the management of patients, especially in problem cases and/or in cases of unfavourable evolution.

> The follow-up was not standardized and homogeneous, but the duration of the follow-up was not the same for all patients.

III- DATA FROM THE LITERATURE :

III-1- Epidemiological study :

III-1-1- Impact :

Despite national and international efforts, tuberculosis continues to be a major global health problem, particularly in the poorest regions [4,5]. Indeed, it is the second leading cause of death from infectious diseases after HIV [4].

Its current recrudescence is partly favoured by HIV infection, the emergence of resistant strains and the important migratory flow of populations on the one hand and the improvement of data collection on the other hand [6].

Although pulmonary localization remains the most common, the frequency of extrapulmonary tuberculosis (EPT) is increasing, with rates ranging from 20 to 60% depending on the series (Table XII).

Table XII: Incidence of lymph node tuberculosis by series

Authors	Country	No. of new cases of tbc/year	Percentage PET
DSSB[2]	Tunisia(2012)	2964	45,2%
Hamzaoui[7]	Morocco(2012)	26000	46%
Peto[8]	USA(2008)	13779	20,4%
Central TB division [9]	India(2015)	260994	61%

In the United States, the proportion of PET increased from 16% in 1993 to 20.4% in 2008, with a preponderance of cervical lymph node location (41%) [8]. In Tunisia, after a decreasing trend, the incidence recognizes since the year 2002 an increasing curve reaching a value of 42/100 000 inhabitants in 2015 [10].

According to WHO, PET accounted for 57.52% of the number of reported TB cases in 2013 [11]. Cervical lymph node localization, which accounts for 70-90% of PET in Tunisia, is experiencing an increasing incidence [12-14] from 2.3 cases /100,000 inhabitants in 1993 to 8.21 cases /100,000 inhabitants in 2013 [15,16]. The highest figures were noted in Greater Tunis (29%), Ben Arous

(8%) and Bizerte (8%) [17].

In our study, the incidence was overall stable with a peak in 2015 at 1.7 times the mean.

III-1-2- Age :

Cervical lymph node tuberculosis does not spare any age group but it is more frequent in adolescents and young adults [20-40 years] (Table XIII). Also in our series, 68% of the patients were aged under 40 years old.

Table XIII: Age distribution

Authors	Country	Year	Number of cases	Average age (years)
Beogo[18]	Burkina Faso	2013	115	31,46
Mahida[19]	Pakistan	2015	46	22
Cho[20]	South Korea	2009	235	35,6
Omura[21]	Japan	2016	38	58,9
Our series	Tunisia	2017	50	34

This preponderance of the condition in the young population implies several problems:

- This is an active population and this pathology will have professional consequences (absenteeism, reduced performance).
- For adolescents in particular, we are frequently confronted with the problems of refusal and poor compliance (in our series, the non-compliers were patients under 20 years of age).
- This last point would be a determining factor in therapeutic failure and the emergence of multi-resistant strains.
- HIV-tuberculosis co-infection, which is frequent in young adults, should be considered in the presence of risky behaviour [22] and/or an atypical evolution of the disease.

III-1-3- Sex :

Several studies support a significant relationship between female gender and PET (Table XIV).

Table XIV Distribution by gender

Author	Mahida[19]	Omura[21]	Fliss[23]	Kermani[24]	Our series
Women (%)	78%	55%	86,9%	30%	52%

An immune and hormonal role, socioeconomic factors and access to care are the most supported theories [25].

In our series, we did not note any gender predominance. This can be explained in part by the military environment in which the study was conducted.

III-2- Predictive factors of lymph node tuberculosis :

It is important for the practitioner to recognize the presumptive factors of a probable tuberculosis involvement, especially in front of an isolated looking adenopathy. This would allow a better early management of patients.

III-2-1- History of tuberculosis :

In the literature, 2-30% of patients treated for lymph node tuberculosis were already affected by the disease [23,26-29]. In this case, it is necessary to systematically search for a multidrug-resistant strain by culture and antibiotic susceptibility testing [1]. In fact, this risk is multiplied by 6 if there is a personal history of tuberculosis and by 2 if there is a family history [30].

In our series, four patients had a personal history of tuberculosis, half of them with a cervical lymph node location.

III-2-2- Tuberculosis test:

Direct contact with a tuberculosis patient is a risk factor for lymph node involvement. A history of tuberculosis in the family has been reported in 12 to 53% depending on the series [31].

It is essentially an intrafamilial contact [32] and/or with a person living in a community [16]. The contaminator is most often a carrier of pulmonary tuberculosis [33].

In our series, the family history of tuberculosis was in 3 cases out of 4 a pulmonary location. This rate is probably underestimated by the fact that the contaminator is unknown (not declared for social considerations or is unaware of it because of lack of screening) and that lymph node tuberculosis may not manifest itself until several years later, making the interrogation often difficult.

In a military environment (living in a community), the notion of contagion is essential. Thus, in the case of any diagnosed tuberculosis, an investigation in the entourage is systematically undertaken. However, we have not found a relationship between the profession, the notion of living in a community and a bad therapeutic evolution.

III-2-3- Raw milk consumption :

The consumption of unpasteurized raw milk and its derivatives seems to play a major role in the transmission of Mycobacterium Bovis, which is responsible for nearly 78% of cases of lymph node tuberculosis in Tunisia, via tuberculous mastitis [34].

It is a habit reported by 33 to 76% of Tunisian patients, particularly those living in rural areas [23,26,28,35]. It was reported by 56% of our patients.

The available data on the contribution of pasteurization have shown a great benefit on public health and an effective reduction of tuberculosis transmission without affecting the nutritional value of this food [36,37].

III-2-4- Co-morbidity :

Tuberculosis infection, particularly in the lymph nodes, is significantly more frequent in cases of immunodepression, whether congenital, acquired or iatrogenic (diabetes, renal failure, cancer, long-term immunosuppressants or corticosteroids, etc.) [38].

Indeed, the defense mechanism against Mycobacterium Tuberculosis Complex involves macrophage and T cell immunity. Thus, any impairment of this mechanism exposes the patient to the risk of a tuberculosis infection, particularly in the lymph nodes (Table XV).

In the study by Gargah et al [39], 25% of renal patients developed cervical lymph node tuberculosis during the first 5 years of hemodialysis.

Table XV Co-morbidity (excluding HIV)

Author	Immunosuppression(%)	Pathology	(%)
Sammoud[16]	9,7%	Diabetes Cancer CRI	5% 4% 10%
Sost[40]	52%	Chronic alcoholism Solid neoplasia Long-term corticosteroid therapy	31% 24% 34%
Our series	8%	Corticosteroid therapy Diabetes	4% 4%

On the other hand, HIV infection increases the risk of developing PET by a factor of 10, which is the leading cause of preventable death in AIDS patients [11].

Cervical lymph nodes represented 46% of all tuberculosis localizations in AIDS patients in the series by Hochedez [22], with a preponderance of disseminated and deep forms. This is why the WHO recommends screening for HIV co-infection in all persons at risk and/or carriers of tuberculosis.

In our series, no patient was known to have AIDS, but only one patient was tested for HIV and returned negative.

III-3- Clinical study :

III-3-1- Circumstances of discovery :

The discovery of adenopathy was the most reported reason for consultation in most series as well as ours. This is due to a recruitment bias, since these were patients consulting an ENT clinic and presenting with apparently isolated adenopathy. The average delay of consultation is variable according to the series, it was 6.9 months in our series and 4 months in Sammoud's series [16]. Patients are only alarmed after several months when they see an insidious evolution of the disease.

III-3-2- Signs of tuberculosis impregnation :

A review of the literature shows that lymph node tuberculosis is rarely associated with general signs [41,42]. Their presence is more frequent in AIDS patients [16,22]; in the series by Wei [43], they were noted in 76% of HIV-positive patients compared with 12% of HIV-negative subjects.

According to the Maghreb report on cervical lymph node tuberculosis [17], a search for other tuberculosis sites and HIV co-infection was recommended when there was at least one clinical sign of tuberculosis impregnation.

In our series, 38% of patients reported general signs. Their presence was not correlated with more severe forms of the disease.

III-3-3- Physical examination :

S All cervical lymph nodes can be affected, but as in our study, the jugulocarotid chain seems to be the most affected [24,44,45]. Indeed, the portal of entry of Mycobacterium Bovis would be oral-pharyngeal, the adenopathy representing a satellite lymph node of the chancre of inoculation [46].

J It is often unilateral [31,45,47], affecting a single area in 86% of cases in the series by Sammoud [16].

J At the time of diagnosis, the number of affected adenopathies varies between series as shown in Table XVI.

Table XVI: Percentage of Multiple EPAs by Study

Series	Belakhdhar [35]	Wei [43]	Abid [48]	Park [49]	Our series
Multiple Adp	54%	20,6%	33%	12,3%	68%

The clinical appearance is different depending on the time of the consultation. Adenopathies are initially firm and mobile and evolve, with the progression of the infection, towards fixity, softening and then fistulization [45,50,51]. However, in Tunisia, diagnosis at the fistulization stage seems to regress over the years; this would be due to improved access to care with earlier management (Table XVII).

Table XVII: Diagnosis of fistulization

Authors	Year	Fistulization to the skin (%)
Chahed[17]	2008-2013	11,3%
Belakhdar [35]	1982-2006	10%
AYOUB [52]	1965-1981	39,4%
ENNOURI [53]	1973-1987	16%
Our series	2009-2016	6%

In practical terms, these data should be taken into consideration:

- Multiple and bilateral adenopathies are in favor of *Mycobacterium Tuberculosis* involvement. Unilateral involvement is in favor of the responsibility of atypical mycobacteria [54].
- Therapeutically, Wei [43] concludes that bilateral involvement is more correlated with treatment failure and recommends more prolonged treatment. Also in our study, the presence of multiple or bilateral adenopathies was associated with failure and difficult management.
- Fistulization is also considered a factor of poor response to treatment and would be a formal indication for surgery [53,55].

III-3-4- Additional examinations :

III-3-4-1- Cervical ultrasound :

Under experienced hands, ultrasound can provide etiological orientation of a lymph node tuberculosis.

Tuberculous adenitis can have different aspects. However, the diagnosis should be made in the presence of a cluster of hypoechoic adenopathies [56] with the presence of intra-lesional necrosis or hyperechoic structures, cystic transformation and blurred boundaries of the adenopathy in relation to peri-adenitis [57,58]. Calcifications may be noted at a late stage [58,59]. With a rate of 76%, the hypoechoic aspect was the most common in the Tunisian multicenter study [17]; necrosis was noted in 42% of cases. Our results were similar.

There is no consensus on the frequency of ultrasound monitoring. Indeed, the presence of residual adenopathy at the end of treatment (noted in up to 41% of cases) does not necessarily mean persistence of the infection [17,60]. Imaging is conditioned by the clinical evolution.

III-3-4-2- Chest X-ray :

In our series, no parenchymal or pleural lesions were found on the routinely performed chest radiograph.

Although rarely described [12,47], the isolation of *Mycobacterium Tuberculosis* in 21% of cases of lymph node tuberculosis in Tunisia [2] makes it necessary to search for an asymptomatic pulmonary localization [29].

III-3-4-3- Other radiological investigations :

- Cervical computed tomography (CT) allows a study of the number and relationships of adenopathies. It is of interest for the exploration of deep lymph node groups and in case of recurrence, especially in view of surgical treatment [61]. Without being specific, Vaid [60] describes three scannographic stages through which tuberculous adenitis passes; first it is hypodense with a homogeneous appearance, then central necrosis appears and finally calcified in places.

- Some authors recommend systematically performing an abdominal ultrasound examination, as *Mycobacterium Bovis* is also responsible for abdominal lymph node tuberculosis, with the possibility of an association of the two localizations [2,62]. However Makni [63] reports a normal examination in 2/3 of cases.

III-4- Diagnostic confirmation :

- ❖ Formerly represented by the tuberculin intradermal reaction, the interpretation of which is sometimes delicate, several immunological tests are currently available. Quantiferon-TB and TSPOT-TB assess, by blood sampling, the secretion of interferon by T lymphocytes in response to one of the specific antigens of *Mycobacterium Tuberculosis*. Their specificity is 97 to 100% with no interference with BCG vaccination and a 24-hour reading [16,64]. Their main drawback is their high cost and moderate sensitivity in immunocompromised patients (30-40%). In our series, despite its recent availability in the hospital, we did not use Quantiferon-TB probably due to lack of practice.

- ❖ Node cytopuncture with bacteriological study has a preponderant place in the diagnosis of tuberculosis, especially in endemic countries where the difficulty of access to care makes it easier to resort to cytopuncture at a lower cost [4]. The rate of confirmation by cytology is however different according to the series; it was 27% in the series of Marrakchi [32], and 71% in the series of Ilgazli [38].

- ❖ Anatomopathological study on lymph node biopsy is however the gold standard in the diagnosis of the disease with a specificity of 90 to 100% [65,66]. It is an invasive examination with a significant cost and aesthetic consequences. In this context, ultrasound-guided trocar biopsy under local anaesthesia may be an interesting alternative, guaranteeing equivalent sensitivity with lower cost and no sequelae [67].

- The final diagnosis is based on the detection of M. Tuberculosis, which remains difficult due to the paucibacillary nature of lymph node tuberculosis.

The development of rapid diagnostic methods has shortened the time required for classical cultures on solid media [16], from 10 to 15 days in the case of cultures on liquid media to less than 48 hours in the case of molecular biology techniques with the possibility of direct identification of species and detection of drug resistance by PCR and GeneXpert [68,69].

Our study points out the very low contribution of bacteriology and especially of BK culture in our hospital compared to the different series.

III-5- Treatment :

The treatment of lymph node tuberculosis is primarily medical. It must be started as soon as the diagnosis is certain.

It is essential that the patient be informed:

- The goals of the treatment and its estimated duration.
- The importance of good compliance and regular monitoring.
- Possible side effects that should be reported to your doctor.

III-5-1- Antibiotic therapy against tuberculosis:

The medical treatment of lymph node tuberculosis is in principle identical to that of the pulmonary form [70]. It is based on the combination of first-line anti-tuberculosis drugs containing at least two major anti-tuberculosis drugs which are Isoniazid (INH) and Rifampicin (RMP).

In accordance with WHO recommendations, the use of ADFs has become systematic in Tunisia since July 2009. The goals of the marketing of these combinations are [71-73]:

- Reduce prescribing errors.
- Improve compliance by reducing the number of tablets to be taken.
- To limit the risk of selection of resistant strains by guaranteeing a synergistic intake of the different molecules.

These fixed-dose combinations are available in several forms of two or more anti-tuberculosis drugs [72] (Table XVIII).

Table XVIII: Presentation of ADFs available in Tunisia

Fixed dose combinationsSubmission	(Dosage)
HRZE	(R 150 mg + H 75 mg + Z 400 mg + E 275 mg)
HR	(R 150 mg + H 75 mg)

The administration of anti-tuberculosis drugs follows certain rules:

- Take the total dose daily and as a single dose.
- Taken on an empty stomach to optimize absorption of isoniazid and rifampin.
- If the patient appears uncooperative, direct supervision of the treatment during the first period is best done in a hospital setting.
- Therefore, any practitioner following up these patients must be aware of the potential side effects of anti-tuberculosis drugs (Annex 2).

III-5-2- Pre-therapeutic assessment :

Before choosing a treatment protocol, a workup is necessary to eliminate a possible contraindication to one of the antibiotics and to provide a reference workup for follow-up during treatment [74]. This assessment includes:

- A clinical examination: weight measurement, search for pathological history and current treatment.

- A blood test including:

- A blood count (CBC).
- Transaminase assay for INH toxicity and MTR.
- The study of renal function and uricemia for PZA toxicity.

- An ophthalmological examination: with study of the visual field, colour vision, visual acuity and fundus. This test looks for an abnormality that would contraindicate the prescription of Ethambutol (ETB). However, in recent studies, several authors recommend keeping ADF with close clinical monitoring every 15 days for the first two months [75].

In our series, we opted for this approach. Thus, among four initial dyschromatopsias, only one was aggravated under HRZE.

- An acetylation test: Its purpose is to identify slow acetylators in order to adapt the dose of INH [76]. Its systematic performance is currently discussed [77].

In practice, this test is increasingly reserved for patients with a history of liver disease or known neurological disorders [78].

Acetylation testing was not routinely performed in our patients. Those who required dose adjustment with a switch to the dissociated form were excluded from the study.

- It should be remembered that since streptomycin is no longer a first-line anti-tuberculosis drug, audiometry is no longer a routine part of the pre-treatment assessment, especially if a decision has been made to start a DSA [79].

In our series, 24 patients were excluded from the study because of a contraindication to the use of ADF (32% of the cases diagnosed). This rate is comparable to that reported in the Tunisian multicenter study on cervical lymph node tuberculosis [17] with 28% of the cases having been put on dissociated anti-tuberculosis drugs due to the presence of abnormalities in the pre-treatment work-up.

III-5-3- Duration of treatment

The WHO recommends a classic two-phase treatment regimen [15,70]:

Initial (intensive) **phase:** combining the 4 first-line anti-tuberculosis drugs in a combined form (HRZE). It lasts 2 months and aims at the rapid destruction of bacilli as well as the prevention of the selection of resistant colonies.

Consolidation phase: combines the two major anti-tuberculosis drugs, isoniazid and rifampicin (HR), for a period of four months to eliminate the remaining bacilli and sterilize the lesions.

However, the literature review did not find a consensus or quality studies concluding on an optimal duration of treatment for lymph node tuberculosis.

Thus, despite the recommendations of the WHO, those of various international organizations in the USA (Centers for Disease Control and Prevention, Infectious Diseases Society of America) and in France (Conseil Supérieur d'Hygiène Publique, Société de Pneumologie de Langue Française) judging that a total duration of treatment of six months is sufficient in the majority of situations [73,80-83], this duration is only rarely respected and the majority of practitioners treated lymph node tuberculosis for a much longer period. The latter was 9.8 ± 4.6 months in the Ben Brahim series [84] and 12.8 months in the Sammoud series [16]. In our series, the average duration of treatment was 9.1 months.

The duration of the intensive phase has been adopted by most of the series, including Tunisian ones [16,84-86], but the duration of consolidation was longer than that recommended by the WHO. We extended the first phase to 3 or 4 months in the case of noncompliance with the treatment with or without paradoxical reaction and we shortened it to 1 month in the case of worsening dyschromatopsia with a change in the therapeutic protocol in two cases.

A review of the literature reveals two attitudes: a minimalist one recommending 6 months and a maximalist one recommending at least 9 months of treatment. Both attitudes are in fact defensible given that :

- Prolonged treatment means more frequent monitoring and a significant cost, as well as greater toxicity and a frequent drop in adherence to treatment [87].
- However, a short duration of treatment may not be sufficient to sterilize the tuberculosis focus because of the limited diffusion of anti-tuberculosis drugs in the lymphoid tissue, especially as the infiltrating nature of the adenopathies rarely allows a complete lymph node evacuation.

Most practitioners, faced with the persistence of clinically significant adenopathy even after 9 months of treatment and for fear of failure, support the need for a prolonged prescription in PET.

4- Nevertheless, the reflection that arises is that since *Mycobacterium Bovis* (responsible for 78% of cases of lymph node tuberculosis in Tunisia) is naturally resistant to pyrazinamide [15,34], we find ourselves with an intensive phase really reduced to a two-month triple therapy.
Thus, some teams recommend extending the duration of ethambutol prescription from 1 to 4 months to accumulate 3 to 6 months of triple therapy [16].

III-5-4- Place of surgery in the treatment of lymph node tuberculosis :

The contribution of surgery in the positive diagnosis of lymph node tuberculosis compared to cytopuncture has been widely documented in the literature [17,22,29]. However, its place in the actual treatment of the condition remains controversial in the face of an infectious pathology supposed to be medically curable with cure rates that are most often satisfactory.

J Apart from a questionable clinical and paraclinical presentation that raises suspicion of malignancy or a significant paradoxical reaction, supporters of a surgical treatment component indicate an operative procedure whenever [24,53,55]:

- The lymph node mass is too large or calcified and medical treatment is not expected to be sufficient due to low diffusion of anti-tuberculosis drugs in the lymph node tissue.
- There is a cold abscess or skin fistulization, a common cause of failure.
- In spite of a well-conducted medical treatment, significant lymph node remnants persist with a cytopunction isolating BK.

J For other authors, surgery is reserved for forms that are resistant to medical treatment [88]:

- The appearance of lymph nodes under treatment.
- Lack of response to treatment (persistence of residual adenopathy despite well-conducted medical treatment).
- The increase in lymph node volume after 3 months of well-conducted treatment including late paradoxical reactions.
- A lymph node recurrence after a well conducted medical treatment.

Ben Brahim [84] concluded that surgery did not improve the cure rate of his patients but it did significantly shorten the duration of medical treatment (8.7 vs 10.6 months, $p = 0.017$).
In the series of Kermani [24], operated patients had significantly lower rates of resistance and recurrence (3.6% and 4.8% respectively) than non-operated patients (53% and 30.7%).

In all cases, the operation should consist, as far as possible, of a true cellulo-lymphadenectomy removing all palpable adenopathies rather than a simple adenectomy [24,47,88].
In our study, surgery was performed for therapeutic purposes in eight cases, including five cases of resistance to treatment, one paradoxical reaction and two cases of recurrence. Five cases were functional lymph node dissection.

J Surgery for tuberculosis is delicate because of the importance of inflammatory phenomena and adhesions to neighbouring structures, making dissection laborious with several possible complications, in particular injury to the thoracic duct, the spinal nerve or the chin ramus of the facial nerve, as well as unsightly scars [36].

However, the use of this therapeutic component is more or less important depending on the series. It seems to be more frequent in the studies conducted in surgical departments, which represents a selection bias that makes it impossible to draw formal conclusions regarding the contribution of surgery in the management of this condition (Table XIX).

Table XIX: Use of surgical treatment

Author	Sammoud [16]	Kermani [24]	Ben moussa [47]	Ben Brahim [84]	Our series
Surgical treatment	5%	96,4%	10%	55%	13%

III-6- Evolution under treatment :

III-6-1- Adverse reactions :

Each anti-tuberculosis drug has its own adverse effects. Their combination may increase some of these effects and become more or less serious. Their incidence varies according to the series (Table XX).

In Sammoud's series [16], 16% of patients required a change in treatment. In our series, we had to change the treatment protocol in 4 cases (8%) following the appearance of side effects under ADF.

Digestive intolerance, hepatotoxicity and skin reactions are the most commonly described adverse events in the literature.

Table XX: Adverse reactions described in the literature

Study	AR (%)	Type of AR	(%)
Gabsi [89]	16%	Digestive intolerance	4,7
		Skin reaction	6,5
		Hepatotoxicity	6,7
		Neuropsychic	1
Lefevre[90]	64,8%	Digestive intolerance	24,3
		Hepatotoxicity	38
		Hyperuricemia	14,2
		NORB	4
		Skin reaction	3,6
		Peripheral neuropathy	4,9
		Arthro-myalgia	13,4
Sahnoun [91]	19,4%	Neurological	32,7
		Skin reaction	32,7
		Hepatic cytolysis	19,23
		Arthralgias	3,8
Our series	52%		

Some authors have tried to compare the incidence of these side effects during treatment with ADF and dissociated anti-tuberculosis drugs. Several authors such as Alshaer et al [92] reported an increase in hepatic and digestive side effects with ADFs, while visual disturbances were more marked with dissociated treatment (p=0.03). Similar results have been reported in other studies [93-95]. This comparison was not conclusive in other series [86].

However, ADFs also pose the problem of handling in the event of a side effect.

When an adverse event occurs, the molecule involved must first be identified:

- The occurrence of an early hepatic manifestation is in favour of the responsibility of isoniazid. When it occurs late, it may be secondary to pyrazinamide or rifampicin. The latter may be accompanied by immune-allergic manifestations . However, a Asymptomatic increase in transaminases only warrants discontinuation of treatment if it exceeds 5 times normal [16,96].
- Digestive disorders are often transient, occurring during the first few weeks of treatment,

and respond well to antiemetics and proton pump inhibitors. In order to keep ADFs, some authors try to administer the dose in two doses with good results [97].

- Allergic manifestations may involve all molecules, ranging from simple skin pruritus to anaphylactic shock. Pyrazinamide and isoniazid are the most frequently incriminated. Treatment should be stopped and reintroduced progressively with a switch to dissociated molecules [16]. These reactions are more frequent in cases of :
  - Of advanced age (by modification of pharmacokinetics).
  - Female and immunocompromised (25% increased risk) [96].
  - Intermittent treatment with repeated administration is the main preventable factor in the occurrence of these events [97].

III-6-2- Evolution of the disease :

Whatever the therapeutic outcome, the declaration of the end of treatment is mandatory with a definition of the patient's status (cure, treatment failure, treatment interrupted...) [75].

III-6-2-1- Paradoxical reaction :

It is manifested by an increase in the size of a pre-existing adenopathy or its fistulization under well-conducted treatment of at least 10 days after an initial improvement [98].

The prevalence of paradoxical reactions varies according to the series, ranging from 2.2% in the series by Sammoud [16] to 23% of cases in the series by Cho [20]. The risk of occurrence is highest between one and three months after the start of treatment [16] and is much higher in patients with AIDS (28% compared with 10% in the absence of AIDS in the series by Breen) [99]. In our series, three patients presented a paradoxical reaction (6%), one of them late.

On the pathophysiological level, a specific immunological mechanism is currently suggested [100].

In fact, in the case of tuberculosis infection, specific T hypo-lymphocytosis develops with a decrease in the secretion of interferon gamma by the monocytes-macrophages. All these abnormalities will be corrected when anti-tuberculosis chemotherapy is started [100,101]. This paradoxical reaction may involve both the adenopathy already affected and other lymph nodes that were not affected at the time of diagnosis, thus explaining the different clinical manifestations.

The therapeutic management of paradoxical reactions is not clearly codified [100,102]. Thus:

- Anti-tuberculosis drugs will be maintained without modification of the dose. Reinforcement with other families of antibiotics will depend on the associated lesions, particularly neurological and/or respiratory. The duration will be prolonged according to the importance of the lesions at the time of the paradoxical reaction [20,100].

- The prescription of corticosteroids is not supported by all authors, since its efficacy has not been demonstrated in comparison with the placebo group [20]. However, others recommend its prescription at a dose of 1 to 2 mg/kg/day for a period of six to eight weeks [103].
- The place of surgery also remains to be defined, but it seems to be justified in the case of bulky adenopathy with vital or functional repercussions on the neighbouring organs [104].

For our cases, only one patient required a flattening because of the non-improvement under drug reinforcement and corticotherapy.

Several studies have identified predictive factors for the development of a significant paradoxical reaction including young age, male gender, initially tender adenopathies, disseminated TB disease and/or severe initial immunosuppression with CD4 counts below 50/mm3 [20,103]. Our patient had a young age (19 years) with tender adenopathies larger than three centimeters.

However, this situation must remain a diagnosis of elimination and it is advisable to first eliminate a therapeutic failure due to poor compliance, an insufficient dose or a resistant strain of mycobacteria [105].

III-6-2-2- Therapeutic failure :

The goal of treatment for active TB is to achieve a permanent cure of the disease while avoiding the development of drug resistance and thus stopping the transmission of the infection.

The definition of treatment failure for lymph node tuberculosis still lacks precision, particularly concerning the date of definition of this status, after which the practitioner must stop treatment and look for a problem of drug resistance [106].

This resistance can be primary but is most often secondary to poorly conducted treatment with several levels of mono, multi or ultra-resistance [16].

In 2013, globally, it is estimated that 3.5% of new reported cases and 20% of previously treated cases carry multidrug-resistant bacilli. In Tunisia the number of reported new cases of multidrug resistant tuberculosis was 730 cases [11].

Rapid diagnostic methods such as the isothermal molecular ring test, reverse hybridization strips, GeneXpert and Xpert Ultra, provide a result within hours, ensuring reliable and early detection of resistance in patients receiving an inadequate initial regimen.

In practice, in the event of a therapeutic failure with a positive result for one of these tests, a conventional antibiotic susceptibility test must be performed, which is the only reference test for confirming resistance [107].

Management, which is not standardized, will be carried out by experts in a specialized service with a combination of five or six drugs. The duration of treatment varies, but is on average 2 years [10,107].

Recent studies recommend shortening the course to 9 months with reinforcement of the combination of seven antibiotics during the attack period. Following this protocol, Van Deun [108], reports a cure rate of 87.9% with better compliance and lower cost.

In our series, the failure rate for medical treatment was 13%. Due to the unavailability of an antibiogram, a modification of the antibiotic therapy was recommended in collaboration with the infectious diseases physicians.

It should be noted that several comparative studies have concluded that the introduction of ADFs did not significantly contribute to a decrease in the rate of resistance and consequently to a decrease in failure rates [86,92].

III-6-2-3- Relapse :

The rate of recurrence or relapse of lymph node tuberculosis varies between series (Table XXI).

Table XXI: Recurrence rates by series

Author	Kermani[24]	Gabsi [89]	Ben Brahim[84]	Our series
Recidivism (%)	4,4%	2,2%	2%	4%

Reducing failure and relapse rates was one of the most important goals of the WHO in introducing ADFs. However, comparative studies between ADF and dissociated forms have not found any significant difference in terms of improved treatment outcomes [15,86]. On the contrary, in a meta-analysis conducted in 2013 including 29 studies including 15 randomized controlled trials, the authors concluded that patients treated with ADFs had the highest recurrence rates with a mean relative risk of 1.28 [109].

However, relapse is not always synonymous with therapeutic failure. It may be due to reinfection of the patient or a paradoxical reaction at a relatively late stage [9,22]. In these cases, surgical management is still recommended by almost all authors [16,47,55].

The aim of the surgery is twofold; firstly, bacteriological diagnosis by allowing isolation of the germ and detection of any resistance via the culture of the lymph node crush, and secondly, therapeutic, by removing the lymph node, to adapt the therapeutic protocol and reduce the duration of the treatment [16,89].

In our series, we opted for a functional lymph node removal in one case due to the massive recurrence. However, the bacteriological study with antibiogram was not performed.

III-6-2-4- Healing :

While the criteria for cure are well detailed for pulmonary tuberculosis, they are not yet codified for lymph node tuberculosis. Thus, according to the NTP, a patient is considered cured if he or she does not show any signs of clinical and/or echographic progression [1].

The therapeutic results vary according to the series (Table XXII), but few studies have investigated the contribution of ADF in lymph node tuberculosis.

Table XXII: Cure rates for lymph node TB

Author	Sammoud [16]	Ben Safta [86]	Gabsi [89]	Lienhardt [110]	Our series
Cure rate	68,1%	73,7%	97,7%	93,9%	87%

Although clinical cure cannot be confirmed, various studies [111,112] have concluded that only a small number of patients will have a complete, radiologically attested disappearance of their adenopathies at the end of treatment.

Thus, several authors question the need for ultrasound monitoring and recommend it rather at the end of the treatment and later to detect a possible evolutionary recovery [112].

The new molecules recently put on the market, in addition to the programmes set up by the WHO and the national anti-tuberculosis programmes, give hope for an improvement in therapeutic results with a lower rate of iatrogenic complications and better tolerance for the patient.

III-7- Special cases :

- Pregnancy is not a contraindication to the treatment of tuberculosis, it is a therapeutic emergency.

In principle, the standard treatment is applicable, but the use of pyrazinamide is discussed because the absence of teratogenic effects has not been formally demonstrated [113]. However, international bodies such as the WHO and the International Union Against

Tuberculosis recommend the use of pyrazinamide, with the possibility of keeping the combined form of treatment [114].

If pyrazinamide is excluded, as recommended by the Maghreb consensus [17], the dual therapy phase should be extended to an average of 7 months.

In our series, we opted for a therapeutic interruption of the pregnancy during the first month. Two were beyond six months of treatment, the malformative risk was considered low and they continued their dual therapy (HR) as normal.

- The discovery of immunosuppression does not contraindicate the combined treatment and the same therapeutic protocol is recommended. However, if the immunosuppression (systemic disease,...) is discovered at the same time as the tuberculosis, the anti-tuberculosis treatment must precede the immunosuppressive treatment by two weeks [16].

- In case of associated pulmonary involvement, the germ incriminated is rather Mycobacterium Tuberculosis. The evolution of lymph node involvement is not influenced by that of the lung and no change in the therapeutic protocol is recommended [17].

III-8- Factors of bad evolution :

Several studies have looked at the factors that contribute to the poor outcome of tuberculosis during treatment (Table XXIII).

- Knowledge of the different factors predicting a bad evolution would allow the clinician to plan an adapted therapeutic course of action (duration of treatment, need for surgery, combination of other anti-tuberculosis drugs...) and to discuss it with the patient from the beginning.

Table XXIII: Factors for poor outcome according to different studies

Author	Country (year)	Problem patients (%)	Factors of poor evolution
Cho[20]	Korea (2009)	10 (4,25%)	Inflammatory signs of PDA Male Young age Immunosuppression
Misombo-K [26]	Congo (2016)	73 (34%)	Non-adherence to treatment History of multidrug-resistant TB Low socio-economic level
Wei[45]	Japan (2009)	6 (6,8%)	Low BMI and malnutrition Bilateral adenopathy Immunosuppression Non-compliance Low socioeconomic level
Chang[115]	China (2004)	113 (0,9%)	Weight < 50 Kg Immunosuppression: diabetes and HIV Association of gg TB and pulmonary TB Treatment compliance
Law[116]	Japan (2008)	156 (14,7%)	Young age Low socio-economic level Frequent travel
Our study	Tunisia (2017)	11 (22%)	Young age, female sex History of TBC Bilateral adenopathy, size >3 cm Necrotic appearance of the adenopathy Adherence to the vascular axis of the neck

After a review of the literature, it seems that poor socio-economic conditions, malnutrition, immunosuppression and non-adherence (due to lack of means and/or availability of treatment) are the most common factors for an unfavourable evolution with a higher risk of therapeutic failure. Thus, the management of tuberculosis disease must involve comprehensive management of the patient both in terms of prevention and cure.

4- **At the end of our study**, we have tried to propose a therapeutic attitude to cervical adenopathy of tuberculous origin. In our opinion, this approach should take into account not only the diagnosis but also the patient's profile, clinical data, bacteriological data (if not available, by orientation of the interview and clinical data), and the evolution under treatment (Figure 12).

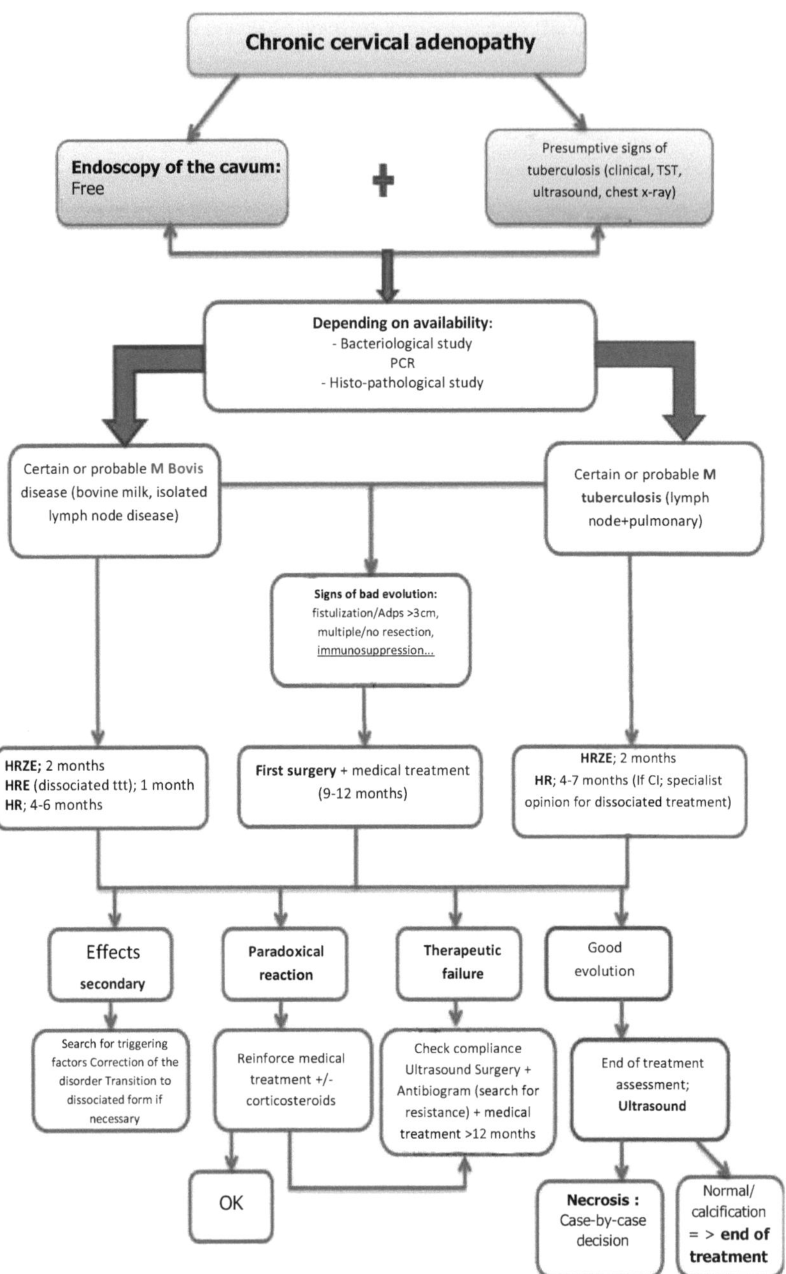

Figure 12: Management of cervical lymph node TB

IV- FUTURE STRATEGIES FOR TUBERCULOSIS CONTROL :

Ending TB is the goal of the WHO's TB strategy and is a target of its Sustainable Development Goals for 2035 [16]. Achieving this goal requires efforts at several levels. Thus, in addition to the strategies already deployed, WHO is working on:

- Strengthening diagnostic and laboratory capabilities :

- Since its first introduction in 2010, the use of the Xpert MTB/RIF rapid test, which is highly recommended by the WHO, has increased significantly. Its cost-effectiveness would be more marked in cases of suspected resistant tuberculosis or in AIDS patients.
- In Tunisia, the need to isolate the germ responsible for the lymph node location is emphasized, which will have important therapeutic consequences.

- Action against TB-HIV co-epidemia :

- WHO estimates that 12% of TB patients worldwide are also HIV positive. Mortality due to TB-HIV co-infection, however, fell by 32% between 2004 and 2014.
- This has largely been achieved through the wider prescription of isoniazid prevention in AIDS patients and the widespread screening of TB patients for HIV infection.

- Research and development :

- In the field of diagnostic tools, tests based on molecular techniques are the most advanced.
- A new generation cartridge called Xpert Ultra to replace the Xpert MTB/RIF cartridge is being developed to replace conventional culture as the primary diagnostic tool for TB at the point of care using a smaller and less expensive device.
- Nine new anti-tuberculosis drugs targeting mainly resistant forms are in advanced stages of clinical trials (bedaquiline, delamanid, linezolid, PBTZ169, pretomanid, Q203, rifapentine and sutezolid).
- Several new treatment regimens are also in advanced stages of testing (in highly endemic countries) with encouraging preliminary results.
- Research, some of it in clinical trials, is under way to develop truly effective TB vaccines that can protect both those already infected and those who are not. The focus has shifted from children to adolescents and adults.

- Educating the population and improving access to care :

- The fight against risk factors, in particular malnutrition, by improving living conditions.
- Early treatment of patients by facilitating access to care and making anti-tuberculosis treatment available.
- Strengthening animal health control measures to interrupt the chain of transmission of animal TB.
- Legislation on the obligation to pasteurise milk and milk products.

- Raising public awareness of the importance of consuming pasteurized dairy products (media, field work, especially in rural areas).

CONCLUSIONS

Despite all the national and international efforts, tuberculosis continues to be a global health problem and studies point to a reappearance of its incidence, especially in its cervical lymph node form, which is the main extra-pulmonary location of the disease.

The insidious nature of the disease, the absence of specific signs and the unavailability of rapid and reliable diagnostic tests often make diagnosis late. Added to these difficulties is the absence of a consensus on the therapeutic protocol, the duration of treatment and follow-up.

In recent years, in order to improve therapeutic results with better tolerance of treatment, the WHO has recommended the prescription of ADFs as a first-line treatment. However, there are still many questions about their efficacy and cost-effectiveness that are raised by practitioners.

Through a retrospective study conducted at the ENT department of the Military Hospital of Tunis during the period from July 2009 to May 2016, we proposed to evaluate the therapeutic results of adult patients treated with the combined form of anti-tuberculosis drugs and to identify the problems related to their use.

We collected 50 patients with a mean age of 34 years. Fifty percent were young adults without gender predominance.

The majority of the patients belonged to a middle class. The notion of living in a community was noted in 14% of cases. BCG vaccination status was specified in only 20 patients (14 of whom were correctly vaccinated) and the consumption of unpasteurized dairy products was reported in 56% of cases.

Four patients had a history of treated tuberculosis (8%), two of which were lymph node, one pulmonary and one digestive. The notion of immunodepression was noted in 4 cases, two of which were on long-term corticosteroid therapy.

All patients consulted because of the finding of cervical swelling associated with general signs in 19 cases.

Sectors III (50%) and II (36%) were the most affected. Adenopathies were bilateral in 18 cases with a mean size of 2.9 cm.

Fistulization to the skin was found in 10% of patients.

On ultrasound, the adenopathies were multiple (80%), hypoechoic (47%) and necrotic (41%). Disseminated involvement was revealed on abdominal-pelvic CT.

The diagnosis of lymph node tuberculosis was confirmed by histological evidence in all patients. A nasopharyngeal tuberculosis location was associated in two cases.

Prior to medical treatment, all our patients underwent a pre-therapeutic assessment revealing dyschromatopsia in 4 cases. A close clinical control during the first two months was recommended with HRZE.

The usual treatment regimen was two months of quadruple therapy (HRZE) followed by six to seven months of dual therapy (HR) with regular clinical and biological follow-up and ultrasound at the end of the treatment. The duration of the quadritherapy was shortened to 1 month in 3 cases due to the appearance of side effects and extended to 3 or 4 months in 3 cases due to non-compliance or a secondary increase in the size of adenopathies.

The average duration of treatment was 9.1 months. It was more than 9 months in 30% of cases and more than 12 months in 4 cases. Eighty percent of patients were compliant.

Under HRZE, 11 patients presented one or more side effects; digestive disorders were the most reported (34%). More serious were visual complications (10%) including one case of NORB followed by intolerance to isoniazid or rifampicin (2 cases). During dual HR therapy, 19 patients experienced adverse events including significant cytolysis and allergy to rifampicin. In total, a switch to the dissociated form was recommended in four cases: 2 during quadruple therapy and 2 during dual therapy.

At the end of the treatment and based on clinical and radiological criteria, 87% of patients were declared cured.

The failure rate in our series was 13%. These cases were treated in collaboration with the infectious diseases department. A combination of other anti-tuberculosis molecules, corticosteroid therapy and/or complementary surgery was recommended with a prolongation of the treatment duration.

The role of surgery is still controversial. Surgical treatment was performed in six cases, including one case of late paradoxical reaction with fistulization. In four cases, the procedure was a functional evacuation.

Two patients had a histologically confirmed relapse after 6 and 12 months of clinical remission.

In our series, young age, female gender, multiple, bilateral adenopathies larger than 3cm with liquefied appearance on ultrasound were the factors associated with poor outcome in our patients.

At the end of this work and after review of the literature, it appears that despite the new therapeutic procedures, lymph node tuberculosis continues to represent a challenge in its diagnosis and therapeutic management.

The introduction of ADFs was based on the hope of minimizing prescribing errors, improving compliance and ensuring the synergistic effect of the different antibiotics. However, these goals do not seem to be achieved according to most authors. They report an increase in adverse effects and relapses with difficulty in adapting doses when necessary. In addition, in our country, the non-availability of all the combined forms obliges the practitioner to frequently switch to the classical dissociated forms.

It is obvious that more needs to be done in terms of prevention. Thus, we insist on the importance of raising the awareness of consumers and professionals regarding the pasteurization of dairy products and of collaborating with veterinarians (to reduce the infestation of the herd and the transmission of bovine tuberculosis).

On the other hand, it is necessary to improve the access to care and the generalization of rapid and reliable diagnostic tests. Finally, a review of the therapeutic protocol in our country seems necessary in view of the frequency of Mycobacterium Bovis making the attack period insufficient.

REFERENCES

1. Direction des Soins de Santé de Base. Guide to the management of tuberculosis in Tunisia. National Tuberculosis Control Program. Tunis: DSSB; 2014.

2. Direction des Soins de Santé de Base. Guide to the management of tuberculosis in Tunisia. National Tuberculosis Control Program. Tunis: DSSB; 2012.

3. Blomberg B, Spinaci S, Fourie B, Laing R. The rationale for recommending fixed-dose combination tablets for treatment of tuberculosis. Bull of Word Health Org. 2001;79(1):61-8.

4. Chouaid C. News in tuberculosis. Rev Mal Respir. 2006;23:80-5.

5. World Health Organization. Global tuberculosis control: surveillance, planning, financing. Switzerland: WHO; 2008.

6. World Health Organization. Global tuberculosis report 2016. Switzerland: WHO; 2016.

7. Hamzaoui G, Amro L, Sajiai H, Serhane H, Moumen N, Ennezari A, et al. Nodal tuberculosis: epidemiological, diagnostic and therapeutic aspects. Pan Afr Med J. 2014;19:157.

8. Peto HM, Pratt RH, Harrington TA, LoBue PA, Armstrong LR. Epidemiology of extrapulmonary tuberculosis in the United States, 1993-2006. Clin Infect Dis. 2009;49:1350-7.

9. Central TB Division Directorate General of Health Services. Ministry of Health and Family Welfare. Annual states report. New Delhi: 2017.

10. World Health Organization. Profile of tuberculosis in Tunisia [Online]. WHO. Available at URL : https://extranet.who.int/sree/Reports?op=Replet&name=%2FWHO_HQ_Report s%2FG2%2FPROD%2FEXT%2FTBCountryProfile&ISO2=TN&LAN=EN&outtype= html.

11. World Health Organization. Tuberculosis [Online]. WHO 2013. Available from URL: http://www.who.int/tb/country/data/profiles/fr/.

12. Tritar F, Daghfous H, Ben Saad S, Slim-Saidi L. Management of multidrug-resistant tuberculosis. Rev Pneumol Clin. 2015;71(2-3):130-9.

13. Barry B, Géhanno P. Ganglionic tuberculosis. Cahier ORL. 1997;32(2):103-6.

14. Khalifa M, Kaabia N, Bahri F, Letaief A, Jemni L. Ganglionic tuberculosis, study of 24 cases observed in a department of Internal Medicine and Infectious Diseases. Maghreb Med. 2002;22(363):250-2.

15. Directorate of Basic Health Care, Ministry of Health, Republic of Tunisia. Study of lymph node tuberculosis in Tunisia. 2015.

16. Sammoud O. Nodal tuberculosis: about 424 cases. [Thesis] Medicine: Tunis; 2015. 139p.

17. Chahed H, Mrabet A, Hariga I, Mbarek C, Tiouiri H. Cervical lymph node tuberculosis in Tunisia: a multicenter study. In: Mbarek C, ed. Cervical lymph node tuberculosis. Tunis: IMPAK; 2015. p. 134-47.

18. Béogo R, Birba NE, Coulibaly TA, Traoré I, Ouoba K. Presentations of tuberculous adenitis of the head and neck at the University Hospital of Bobo- Dioulasso, Burkina Faso. Pan Afr Med J. 2013;15:131.

19. Mahida KH, Akhtar S. Cervical tuberculosis lymphadenitis: experience at tertiary care hospital. Pak J Chest Med. 2015;21(1):10-4.

20. Cho OH, Park KH, Kim T, Song EH, Jang EY, Lee EJ, et al. Paradoxical responses in non-HIV-infected patients with peripheral lymph node tuberculosis. J Infect. 2009;59(1):56-61.

21. Omura S, Nakaya M, Mori A, Oka M, Ito A, Kida W, et al. A clinical review of 38 cases of cervical tuberculous lymphadenitis in Japan- The role of neck dissection. Auris Nasus Larynx. 2016;43(6):672-6.

22. Hochedez P, Zeller V, Truffot C, Ansart S, Caumes E, Tubiana R, et al. Lymph- node tuberculosis in patients infected or not with HIV: general characteristics, clinical presentation, microbiological diagnosis and treatment. Pathol Biol. 2003;51(9):496-502.

23. Fliss M, Meftahi N, Dekhil N, Mhenni B, Ferjaoui M, Rammeh S, et al. Epidemiological, clinical, and bacteriological findings among Tunisian patients with tuberculous cervical lymphadenitis. Int J Clin Exp Pathol. 2016;9(9):9602- 9611.

24. Kermani W, Bouattaya R, Ghammem M, Belakhder M, Ben Ali M, Abdelkafi M, et al. Treatment of cervical lymph node tuberculosis: about 361 cases. J Tun ORL. 2013;28:46-50.

25. Chan-Yeung M, Noertjojo K, Chan SL, Tam CM. Sex differences in tuberculosis in Hong Kong. Int J Tuberc Lung Dis. 2002;6(1):11-8.

26. Smaoui S, Mezghanni MA, Hammami B, Zalila N, Marouane C, Kammoun S, et al. Tuberculosis lymphadenitis in a southeastern region in Tunisia:Epidemiology, clinical features, diagnosis and treatment. Int J Mycobacteriol. 2015;4:196-201.

27. El Bousaadani A, Benbakh M, Zouak A, Eljahd L, Abada Reda A, Rouadi S, et al. Diagnosis and medical-surgical management of cervical lymph node tuberculosis in Morocco: a series of 420 cases. Maghreb Med [Online]. 2015 May [05/06/2017] ;1(226):[38 pages]. Available from URL: http://www.santetropicale.com/revue.asp?revue=mag&id_article=2748&id_numero=226.

28. Abassi H. Management of lymph node tuberculosis culture, typing and antibiogram: about 108 cases. [Thesis] Medicine: Morocco; 2013. 98p.

29. Meddeb R. Cervical lymph node tuberculosis: about 103 cases. [Thesis] Medicine: Tunis; 2004. 117p.

30. Misombo-Kalabela A, Nguefack-Tsague G, Kalla G, Ze E, Diangs K, Panda T, et al. Risk factors for multidrug-resistant tuberculosis in the city of Kinshasa, Democratic Republic of Congo. Pan Afr Med J. 2016;23:157.

31. Berraies A, Bouhaouel W, Snen H, Hedhli A, Ammar J, Hamzaoui A. Results of screening for tuberculosis after tuberculosis contact in 83 children in a pneumo-paediatric department in Tunisia. Rev Mal Respir. 2014;31 Suppl1:S169.

32. Marrakchi C, Maaloul I, Lahiani D, Hammami B, Boudawara T, Zribi M, et al. Diagnosis of peripheral lymph node TB in Tunisia. Med Mal Infect. 2010;40(2):119-22.

33. Bailey WC, Gerald LB, Kimerling ME, Redden D, Brook N, Bruce F, et al. Predictive model to identify positive tuberculosis skin test results during contact investigations. JAMA. 2002;287(8):996-1002.

34. Slim-Saidi L, Gamara D, Messaadi F, Ghariani A, Fourati F, Hili K, et al. A nationwide survey of multidrug resistance among tuberculosis patients in Tunisia. Int J Tuberc Lung Dis. 2012;16

Suppl1:S191.

35. Bellakhdhar M. Cervical lymph node tuberculosis: about 311 cases. [Thesis] Medicine: Sousse; 2008. 124p.

36. Claeys WL, Cardoen S, Daube G, Block JD, Dewettinck K, Dierick K, et al. Raw or heated cow milk consumption: review of risks and benefits. Food Control. 2013;31(1):251-62.

37. Roug A, Perez A, Mazet J, Clifford DL, VanWormer E, Paul G, et al. Comparison of intervention methods for reducing human exposure to Mycobacterium bovis through milk in pastoralist households of Tanzania. Prev Vet Med. 2014;115(3):157-65.

38. Ilgazli A, Boyaci H, Basyigit I, Yildiz F. Extra pulmonary tuberculosis: clinical and epidemiologic spectrum of 636 cases. Arch Med Res. 2004;35(5):435-41.

39. Gargah T, Goucha-Louzir R, Lakhoua MR. Tuberculosis in children undergoing hemodialysis. Int J Nephrol Renovasc Dis. 2010;3:47-50.

40. Sost G, Arvieux C, Cazalets C, Cador B, Delaval P, Michelet C. Factors of immunodepression in tuberculosis patients. Presse Med. 2005;34(6):420-4.

41. Prasad KC, Sreedharan S, Chakravarthy Y, Prasad SC. Tuberculosis in the head and neck: experience in India. J Laryngol Otol. 2007;121(10):979-85.

42. Jha B, Dass A, Nagarkar N, Gupta R, Singhal S. Cervical tuberculous lymphadenopathy: Changing clinical pattern and concepts in management. Postgrad Med J. 2001;77(905):185-7.

43. Wei YF, Liaw YS, Ku SC, Chang YL, Yang PC. Clinical features and predictors of a complicated treatment course in peripheral tuberculous lymphadenitis. J Formos Med Assoc. 2008;107(3):225-31.

44. Hemdani N. Ganglionic tuberculosis. [Thesis] Medicine: Tunis; 2010.

45. Ben Rejeb H. Contribution of lymph node cytopuncture in the diagnosis of tuberculosis. [Thesis] Medicine: Tunis; 2012. 82p.

46. Brodey MV, Zeglin KM, Nayyar S, Degilio M, Rawling RA, Granato PA. Tuberculous Cervical Lymphadenitis. Clin Microbiol Newsl. 2010;32(19):148-50.

47. Ben Moussa N. Cervical lymph node tuberculosis in children: from diagnosis to management about 41 cases. [Thesis] Medicine: Tunis; 2015. 119p.

48. Abid S. Cervical lymph node tuberculosis: about 75 cases. [Thesis] Medicine: Sfax; 2002. 73p.

49. Park KH, Lee MS, Lee SO, Choi SH, Kim YS, Woo JH, et al. Incidence and outcomes of paradoxical lymph node enlargement after anti-tuberculosis therapy in non-HIV patients. J Infect. 2013;67(5):408-15.

50. Mejri Y. Contribution of ultrasound in the diagnosis and follow-up of cervical lymph node tuberculosis. [Thesis] Medicine: Tunis; 2013.

51. Pessey JJ, Rose X, Vergez S. Cervical adenopathy. Encycl Med Chir. (Elsevier Masson, Paris), Otolaryngology, 20870-A-10, 2008, 15p.

52. Ayoub A, Fourati M. Tuberculous cervical adenopathies: about 147 cases. Tunis Med. 1984;62(2):159-62.

53. Ennouri A. Lymph node tuberculosis about 110 cases in Tunisia. Rev Laryngol Otol Rhinol. 1989;110(2):179-81.

54. Muzaffar TM, Shaifuzain AR, Imran Y, Haslina MN. Hematological changes in tuberculosis spondylitis patients at the Hospital University Sains Malaysia. Southeast Asian J Trop Med Public Health. 2008;39(4):686-9.

55. Mani R, Belcadhi M, Harrathi K, Rejeb AB, Benali M, Abdelkefi M, et al. Mycobacterial cervical lymphadenitis: role of surgery. Rev Laryngol Otol Rhinol. 2005;126(2):99-103.

56. Park JH, Kim DW. Sonographic Diagnosis of Tuberculosis Lymphadenitis in the Neck. J Ultrasound Med. 2014;33(9):1619-26.

57. Ahuja A, Ying M, Yuen YH, Metreweli C. Power Doppler Sonography to Differentiate Tuberculous Cervical Lymphadenopathy From Nasopharyngeal Carcinoma. Am J Neuroradiol. 2001;22(4):735-740.

58. Ahuja A, Ying M, Evans R, King W, Metreweli C. The application of ultrasound criteria for malignancy in differentiating tuberculous cervical adenitis from metastatic nasopharyngeal carcinoma. Clin Radiol. 1995;50(6):391-5.

59. Ying M, Ahuja A, Book F. Accuracy of sonographic vascular features in differentiating different causes of cervical lymphadenopathy. Ultrasound Med Biol. 2004;30(4):441-7.

60. Vaid S, Lee YY, Rawat S, Luthra A, Shah D, Ahuja AT. Tuberculosis in the head and neck-a forgotten differential diagnosis. Clin Radiol. 2010;65(1):73-81.

61. Deveci HS, Kule M, Kule ZA, Habesoglu TE. Diagnostic challenges in cervical tuberculous lymphadenitis. North Clin Istanbul. 2016;3(2):150-55.

62. Majoor CJ, Magis-Escurra C, Ingen J, Boeree MJ, Soolingen D. Epidemiology of Mycobacterium bovis Disease in Humans, the Netherlands, 1993-2007. Emerg Infect Dis. 2011;17(3):457-463.

63. Makni F. Ganglionic tuberculosis in children: about 20 observations. [Thesis] Medicine: Sfax; 2012. 153p.

64. Hamzaoui A, Yaalaoui S, Tritar Cherif F, Slim Saidi L, Berraies A. Childhood tuberculosis: a concern of the modern world. Eur Respir Rev. 2014;23(133):278-91.

65. World health organization. Global tuberculosis report 2013. Geneva: WHO; 2013.

66. Hirachand S, Lakhey M, Akhter J, Thapa B. Evaluation of fine needle aspiration cytology of lymph nodes in Kathmandu Medical College, Teaching hospital. Kathmandu Univ Med J. 2009;7(26):139-42.

67. McAllister KA, MacGregor FB. Diagnosis of tuberculosis in the head and neck. J Laryngol Otol. 2011;125(6):603-7.

68. Pahwa R, Hedau S, Jain S, Jain N, Arora VM, Kumar N, et al. Assessment of possible tuberculous lymphadenopathy by PCR compared to non-molecular methods. J Med Microbiol. 2005;54(9):873-8.

69. Derese Y, Hailu E, Assefa T, Bekele Y, Mihret A, Aseffa A, et al. Comparison of PCR with standard culture of fine needle aspiration samples in the diagnosis of tuberculosis lymphadenitis. J Infect Dev Ctries. 2012;6(1):53-7.

70. Lanoix JP, Douadi Y, Borel A, Andrejak C, El Samad Y, Ducroix JP, et al. Treatment of lymph node tuberculosis: from recommendations to practice. Med Mal Infect. 2011;41(2):87-91.

71. World Health organization. Global Tuberculosis report 2014. Geneva: WHO; 2014.

72. Direction des Soins de Santé de Base. Report of the evaluation mission of the national program of tuberculosis control in Tunisia. Tunis: DSSB; 2011.

73. World Health Organization. Guidelines for treatment of tuberculosis: 4th ed. Geneva: WHO; 2010.

74. Dinh A, Perronne C. Clinical and therapeutic aspects of tuberculosis in adults and children. Encycl Med Chir. (Elsevier Masson, Paris), Infectious Diseases, 8038-C-30, 2013, 11p.

75. Nicolet G, Rochat T, Zellweger JP. Treatment of tuberculosis. Forum Med Suisse. 2003;22:506-516.

76. Desnos J, Carbonnelle B, Dubin J. Cervicofacial infections with atypical mycobacteria and lymph node tuberculosis. Ann Otol Laryngol. 1982;99:391-6.

77. Touré A, Cabral M, Diop C, Diene N, Fall M, Dieye AM, et al. Determination of N-acetyltransferase 2 acetylation polymorphism in the Senegalese population by using the caffeine test. Ann Toxicol Anal. 2012;24(3):119-27.

78. Negri L, Le Grusse J, Séraissol P, Lavit M, Houin G, Gandia P. Tuberculosis: interest of isoniazid dosage in the prevention of hepatotoxic effects. Therapie. 2014;69(6):509-16.

79. World Health Organization. Guidelines for treatment of tuberculosis. Geneva: WHO; 2009.

80. Griffith DE, Aksamit T, Brown-Elliott BA, Catanzaro A, Daley C, Gordin F, et al. An official ATS/IDSA statement: diagnosis, treatment, and prevention of nontuberculous mycobacterial diseases. Am J Respir Crit Care Med. 2007;175(4):367-416.

81. Yuen AP, Wong SH, Tam CM, Chan SL, Wei WI, Lau SK. Prospective randomized study of the thrice-weekly six-month and nine-month chemotherapy for cervical tuberculous lymphadenopathy. Otolaryngol Head Neck Surg. 1997;116(2):189-92.

82. Bouchikh S, Stirnemann J, Prendki V, Porcher R, Kesthmand H, Morin AS, et al. Duration of treatment for extrapulmonary tuberculosis: six months or more? Analysis of the TB-INFO database. Rev Med Interne. 2012;33(12):665- 71.

83. Veziris N, Aubry A, Truffot-Pernot C. Arguments about the duration of anti-tuberculosis treatment. Presse Med. 2006;35:1758-64.

84. Ben brahim H, Kooli I, Aouam A, Toumi A, Loussaief C, Koubaa, et al. Diagnostic and therapeutic management of lymph node TB in Tunisia. Pan Afr Med J. 2014;19:211.

85. Menon K, Bem C, Gouldesbrough D, Strachan DR. A clinical review of 128 cases of head and neck tuberculosis presenting over a 10 year period in Bradford. J Laryngol Otol. 2007;121(4):362-8.

86. Ben Safta B, Mehiri N, Kotti A, Toujani S, Ben Salah N, Ouahchi Y, et al. Contribution of fixed-dose combinations (FDCs) of tuberculosis therapy in the treatment of tuberculosis. Tunis Med. 2016;94(7):401-405.

87. Tattevin P. Treatment of tuberculosis in 2007. Med Mal infect. 2007;37(10):617-28.

88. Amman FF, Bani Hani AH, Ghariebeh KI. Tuberculosis of the lymph glands of the neck: a limited role for surgery. Otolaryngol Head Neck Surg. 2003;128(4):576-80.

89. Gabsi A. Cervical lymph node tuberculosis: Clinical study and evaluation of therapeutic results about 501 cases. [Thesis] Medicine: Monastir; 2014.

90. Lefevre B, Revest M, Patrat-Delon S, Piau C, Arvieux C, Tattevin P, et al. Tolerance of anti-tuberculosis treatments in 247 patients. Med Mal Infect. 2014;44(6):14.

91. Sahnoun I, Toujeni S, Mjid M, Akad A, Moamed B, Ben Salah N, et al. Management of short-term side effects (SE) of antituberculosis drugs. Rev Mal Respir. 2015;32:230-231.

92. AlShaer M, Mansour H, Elewa H, Salameh P, Iqbal F. Treatment outcomes of fixed-dose combination versus separate tablet regimens in pulmonary tuberculosis patients with or without diabetes in Qatar. BMC Infect Dis. 2017;17:118.

93. Aouam K, Chaabane A, Loussaïef C, Ben Romdhane F, Boughattas NA, Chakroun M. Adverse effects of anti-tuberculosis drugs: epidemiology, mechanisms and management. Med Mal Infect. 2007;37(5):253-61.

94. Lienhardt C, Cook SV, Burgos M, York-Edwards V, Rigouts L, Anyo G, et al. Efficacy and safety of a 4-Drug fixed-dose combination regimen compared with separate drugs for treatment of pulmonary tuberculosis. The study C randomized controlled trial. JAMA. 2011;305(14):1415-23.

95. Gravendeel JM, Asapa AS, Becx-Bleumink M, Vrakking HA. Preliminary results of an operational field study to compare side effects, complaints and treatment results of a single-drug short-course regimen with a four-drug fixed-dose combination (4FDC) regimen in South Sulawesi, Republic of Indonesia. Tuberculosis (Edinb). 2003;83:183-6.

96. Bouchentouf R, Yasser Z, Benjelloune A, Aitbenasser MA. Hypersensitivity manifestations to antituberculosis drugs. J Fran Viet Pneu. 2011;2(5):4-8.

97. Moubachir H, Ahmed I, Bourkadi JE, Iraqi G. A rare and serious immunoallergic effect of antituberculosis therapy: neutropenia to pyrazinamide. Rev Fr Allergol. 2013;53(6):533-6.

98. Guinchard AC, Pasche P. Cervical tuberculous lymphadenitis and paradoxical reaction: diagnosis and treatment. Rev Med Suisse. 2012;8:1860-5.

99. Breen RA, Smith CJ, Bettinson H, Dart S, Bannister B, Johnson MA, et al. Paradoxical reactions during tuberculosis treatment in patients with and without HIV co-infection. Thorax. 2004;59(8):704-7.

100. Meybeck A, Just N, Nyunga M, Bourahla M, Wallaert B. Efficacy of needle aspiration during a case of paradoxical hypertrophy of tuberculous lymphadenitis. Rev Mal Respir. 2003;20(6):973-7.

101. Hirsch CS, Toossi Z, Othieno C, Johnson JL, Schwander SK, Robertson S, et al. Depressed T-cell interferon-gamma responses in pulmonary tuberculosis: analysis of underlying mechanisms and modulation with therapy. J Infect Dis. 1999;180(6):2069-73.

102. Nataraj G, Kurup S, Pandit A, Mehta P. Correlation of fine needle aspiration cytology, smear and culture in tuberculous lymphadenitis: a prospective study. J Postgrad Med. 2002;48(2):113-116.

103. Kumar R, Prakash M, Jha S. Paradoxical response to chemotherapy in neurotuberculosis. Pediatr Neurosurg. 2006;42(4):214-22.

104. Goussard P, Gie RP, Janson JT, le Roux P, Kling S, Andronikou S, et al. Decompression of Enlarged Mediastinal Lymph Nodes Due to Mycobacterium Tuberculosis Causing Severe Airway Obstruction in Children. Ann Thorac Surg. 2015;99(4):1157-63.

105. Ben Mansour N, El Alani NE. Paradoxical reaction. In: Mbarek C, ed. Cervical lymph node tuberculosis. Tunis: Impak; 2015. p. 94-7.

106. Becerra MC, Freeman J, Bayona J, Shin SS, Kim JY, Furin JJ, et al. Using treatment failure under effective directly observed short course chemotherapy programs to identify patients with multidrug-resistant tuberculosis. Int J Tuberc Lung Dis. 2000;4(2):108-14.

107. World Health Organization. Towards universal access to diagnosis and treatment of multidrug-resistant extensively drug-resistant tuberculosis by 2015. Geneva. WHO; 2011.

108. Van Deun A, Maug AK, Salim MA, Das PK, Saker MR, Daru P, et al. Short, highly effective and inexpensive standardized treatment of multidrug tuberculosis. Am J Respir Crit Care Med. 2010;182(5):684-92.

109. Albanna A, Smith BM, Cowan D, Menzies D. Fixed-dose combination antituberculosis therapy: a systematic review and meta-analysis. Eur Respir J. 2013;42(3):721-32.

110. Lienhardt C, Cook SV, Burgos M, Yorke-Edwards V, Rigouts L, Anyo G, et al. Efficacy and safety of a 4-drug fixed-dose combination regimen compared with separate drugs for treatment of pulmonary tuberculosis: the Study C randomized controlled trial. JAMA. 2011;305(14):1415-23.

111. Ridene I, Ben Salah Y, Daghfous D, Hantous S, Zidi S, Baccouche I et al. Cervical lymph node tuberculosis: ultrasound follow-up [Online]. Société Française de Radiologie [cited 2010/10/29]. Available from URL: http://pe.sfrnet.org/ModuleConsultationPoster/posterDetail.aspx?intIdPoster=4273#ctl00_plhContainerModule_hypSeeCommentAncre.

112. Daghfous H, Mejri Y, Ben Saad S, Kotti A, Kahloul O, Ben Miled, et al. Contribution of cervical ultrasound in the diagnosis and follow-up of cervical lymph node tuberculosis. Tunis Med. 2014;92(01):63.

113. Lessnau KD, Qarah S. Multidrug-resistant tuberculosis during pregnancy: Case report and review of the literature. Chest. 2003;123(3):953-6.

114. Dautzenberg B, Frechet-Jachym M, Maffre JP, Cardot E, Grignet JP. When not to apply the standard treatment for tuberculosis disease? Rev Mal Respir. 2004;21(3):75-97.

115. Chang KC, Leung CC, Yew WW, Ho SC, Tam CM. A nested case-control study on treatment-related risk factors for early relapse of tuberculosis. Am J Respir Crit Care Med. 2004;170(10):1124-30.

116. Law WS, Yew WW, Chiu Leung C, Kam KM, Tam CM, Chan CK, et al. Risk factors for multidrug-resistant tuberculosis in Hong Kong. Int J Tuberc Lung Dis. 2008;12(9):1065-70.

ANNEXES

ANNEX 1:

File no. Name and surname

AgeSexe

OriginAddress

OccupationCommunity Living

Background

Vaccination status (BCG)

ATCD tbc: yes /no Location: TTT followed: Cure declared

ATCD tbc in the family: yes / no

Immunosuppression: DTC in progress Other pathologies

Habits

Consumption of raw dairy products Tobacco Alcohol

Clinical study

CDD Consultation period

Functional signs: Lateral cervical swelling

Signs of tbc impregnation

Other

Clinical examination:

Cervical adenopathy:

- Number
- Location: sector: I / lia / Ilb / III / IV / V / VI
- Side: Right/Left/Bilateral
- Minimum and maximum size (mm)
- Skin appearance over adenopathy: Normal/ Inflammatory/ Fistula Sensitivity
- Consistency Mobility
- Other ganglion chains
- Other locations: ENT Extra-ORL:

Additional examinations:

- Tuberculin test: chest x-ray
- Cervical ultrasound: number/size/laterality/echogenicity/necrosis
- Other: abdominal ultrasound, CT scan.

- BK in sputum:

- Let's quantify:

Diagnostic confirmation:

- Adenectomy Biopsy of the edges of a fistula
- Cytological study: lymph node pellet / lymph node puncture fluid **Pre-therapeutic assessment:**
- Liver function tests: ALT /ASAT / PAL
- CBC: Renal Chemistry Uricemia
- Ophthalmological examination.
- Acetylation test.

Therapeutic protocol:

- Treatment: Quadruple (HRZE): duration Double (HR): total duration
- Compliance with treatment
- Monitoring: Biological

	Initial	1 month	3 months	6 months	9 months	12 months
ASAT/ALAT						
PAL						
Creator/urea						
Uricemia						
Hg/GB/Plq						

Treatment-related adverse events

- Hepatotoxicity - Neurotoxicity - Hematological impairment
- Algodystrophy - Skin allergy
- Digestive - Arthralgia - Hyperuricemia
- Optic neuritis (NORB) - Dyschromatopsia

Evolution:

- Lost and Found - Healing
- Treatment failure - Relapse on discontinuation of treatment
- Node recurrence - Fistulization
- Paradoxical reaction Delay in starting treatment

Surgical treatment

If yes;

- First - Second: cause
- Type of surgery: Functional/selective lymph node removal/ Adenectomy Evacuation of a cold abscess with curettage of its wall
- Final anatomopathological result - Antibiogram
- Modification of medical treatment - total duration of treatment

Cure / Death / Aggravation

ANNEX 2:

Main adverse effects of ADF anti-tuberculosis drugs

Molecule	Undesirable effects
Isoniazid	Liver toxicity, Digestive disorders Allergic skin manifestations, NORB Decreased metabolism of anticonvulsants, epilepsy if overdosed Pancytopenia
Rifampicin	Liver toxicity, Digestive disorders Orange coloration of urine, tears Immediate or delayed hypersensitivity Arthus phenomenon with acute renal failure Increased metabolism of oral contraceptives , sulfonamides hypoglycemic drugs, corticosteroids, VKAs.
Pyrazinamide	Liver toxicity (especially at high doses) Rash, flushing or isolated fever Hyperuricemia, arthralgia
Ethambutol	Dose-dependent vision disorders (CV, colour discrimination, NORB) Allergic skin reactions Hyperuricemia

Therapeutic results of combined treatment of lymph node-cervical tuberculosis

Summary

Introduction:

Cervical lymph node disease remains the most common extrapulmonary tuberculosis (TB) site. Since the introduction of the combined form of anti-tuberculosis drugs, better compliance with treatment and better therapeutic results are estimated.

The objective of this work was to evaluate the therapeutic results of patients treated with the combined form of anti-tuberculosis drugs and to identify the problems associated with the use of this form.

Methods:

This was a retrospective study of patients with TB treated with the combined form of anti-tuberculosis drugs according to the strategy recommended by the national tuberculosis control programme. A minimum follow-up time of 6 months after the end of treatment was required.

Results:

Fifty patients were included in the study. The duration of the quadritherapy was shortened to 1 month in 3 cases and extended to 3 or 4 months in 1 and 2 cases respectively. The total duration of medical treatment varied from 6 to 18 months with a good compliance rate of 80%.

Digestive disorders were the most commonly reported adverse events. Elsewhere, visual disturbances such as dyschromatopsia and retrobullary optic neuropathy, liver cytolysis and cholestasis were reported. Allergic manifestations related to intolerance to isoniazid or rifampicin were noted in one case each. Three patients showed a paradoxical reaction. In total, a switch to the dissociated form was recommended in four cases.

The treatment failure rate was 13% with surgical management in 8 cases including 2 cases for recurrence. After healing, two patients presented a recurrence.

The main factors that appeared to be associated with poor outcome were female gender, history of tuberculosis, bilateral adenopathy, necrotic appearance, size greater than 3 cm and/or adherence to the vascular axis.

Conclusion:

There is no consensus on the treatment of cervical lymph node TB. No study has proven the superiority of the combined form over the dissociated form in terms of cure and adverse effects.

Therapeutic results of combined drug treatment of cervical lymph node tuberculosisAbstract

Background :

Cervical lymph node tuberculosis remains the most common localization of extrapulmonary tuberculosis.One of the main advantages of fixed drug combinations is that patients have to take considerably fewer pills, thus making treatment easier, aiding adherence and eliminating the risk of developing drug resistance attributable to selective drug intake.

This study aimed to assess the therapeutic results of patients treated by combined drug and indicate the limits of this regimen.

Methods:

We retrospectively reviewed patients who presented with cervical lymph node tuberculosis and received the fixed-dose drug combination.

Our therapeutic protocol was based on the national tuberculosis control program recommendations as one further step to ensure adequate treatment of patients. A feed-back of 6 months was required.

Results :

There were 50 patients. The duration of daily quadruple anti-tuberculous drugs has been reduced to 1 month in 3 cases, prolonged to 3 months in 1 case and to 4 months in 2 cases.

Total treatment duration stretched from 6 to 18 months. Eighty per cent of patients were adherent to their treatment.

Gastrointestinal disorders were the most common adverse events. Elsewhere, we noticed visual disorders such as dyschromatopsia and optic neuritis, hepatotoxicity and cholestasis. Two patients developed allergic skin reaction to both isoniazid and rifampicin. Three patients developed a paradoxal response.

In total, a change to the dissociated form was recommended in 4 cases and 6 patients (13%) had to undergo a surgical intervention because of treatment failure.Lymph nodes recurrence was reported in 2 cases (4%).

Female patients, history of tuberculosis, bilateral cervical nodal distribution, necrotic morphology, size superior to 3 cm and adhesion to the vascular axis may be considered as a predictor of a complicated treatment course.

Conclusion:

There is still no consensus on the regimen of antimicrobial treatment of cervical Lymph node tuberculosis.

There is no evidence of superiority of fixed-dose combination of anti-tuberculosis therapy over separate administration in terms of treatment effectiveness.

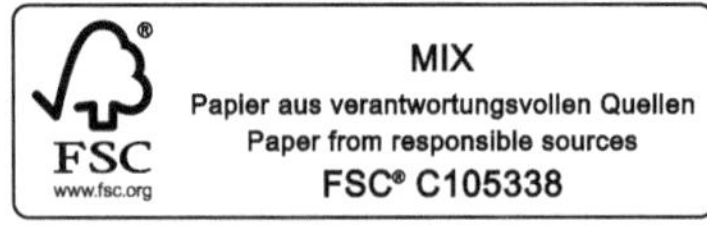

Printed by Books on Demand GmbH, Norderstedt / Germany